Mentally Disordered Offenders

Mentally disordered offenders present particular problems in our society: how do we get the balance right between sympathy towards their illness and genuine worries about their offending behaviour? What do we do for – and about – people who have been released from prison yet who we suspect continue to pose risks to the safety of others?

Mentally Disordered Offenders presses the case for better health care of mentally disturbed law breakers, and the need to divert them from unnecessary imprisonment. With specialist contributors from criminology, criminal justice, social work, probation practice and the law, the book stresses the importance of professional cooperation in community-based services, whilst acknowledging the psychologically demanding nature of working with mentally disordered people.

Mentally Disordered Offenders marks the seventieth birthday of Herschel Prins, whose work has been so influential in this area, and will be an invaluable resource for all those involved in the criminal justice, social welfare, legal and mental health professions.

David Webb is Dean of the Faculty of Economics and Social Science at Nottingham Trent University. **Robert Harris** is Professor in the Department of Politics and Asian Studies at the University of Hull.

Contributors: Philip Bean; Louis Blom-Cooper; Paul Cavadino; Daniel Grant; Jill Peay; Judith Pitchers; Michael Preston-Shoot; John Wood.

Mentally Disordered Offenders

Managing people nobody owns

Edited by David Webb and
Robert Harris

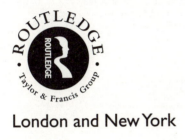

London and New York

First published 1999 by Routledge
11 New Fetter Lane, London EC4P 4EE

Simultaneously published in the USA and Canada
by Routledge
29 West 35th Street, New York, NY 10001

Routledge is an imprint of the Taylor & Francis Group

© 1999 David Webb and Robert Harris, selection and editorial matter;
individual chapters, the contributors

Typeset in Times by
Keystroke, Jacaranda Lodge, Wolverhampton
Printed and bound in Great Britain by
MPG Books Ltd, Bodmin

British Library Cataloguing in Publication Data
A catalogue record for this book is available
from the British Library

Library of Congress Cataloging in Publication Data
Mentally disordered offenders: managing people nobody owns/edited
    by David Webb and Robert Harris.
        p.   cm.
    Includes bibliographical references.
    1. Mentally handicapped offenders—Services for—United States.
    2. Mentally handicapped offenders—Care—United States. 3. Mentally
    handicapped offenders—Mental health services—United States.
    4. Psychiatric social work—United States. I. Webb, David, 1946– .
    II. Harris, Robert, 1947– .
    HV6791.M43   1999
    362.2′086′927—dc21   98-53740

ISBN 0–415–18009–0 (hbk)
ISBN 0–415–18010–4 (pbk)

Contents

List of contributors   ix
Preface   xi

Introduction   1
DAVID WEBB AND ROBERT HARRIS

1 **Mental disorder and social order: underlying themes in
   crime management**   10
   ROBERT HARRIS

   Mental disorder and criminality: some boundary issues 11
   Order, disorder and all stations in between 14
   Justice and order 18
   In conclusion 21
   Notes 24
   References 24

2 **Public Inquiries in mental health (with particular reference
   to the Blackwood case at Broadmoor and the
   patient-complaints of Ashworth Hospital)**   27
   LOUIS BLOM-COOPER

   Preamble 27
   Public and private inquiries 27
   Public or private? 33
   Note 36
   References 36

3 **The police and the mentally disordered in the community** 38
PHILIP BEAN

Legal and procedural objections 39
Police and police stations 40
Recording Section 136 and police procedures 44
Arrangements for treatment and care 46
Future developments 47
Conclusions 49
Notes 50
References 51

4 **Diverting mentally disordered offenders from custody** 53
PAUL CAVADINO

How many mentally disordered prisoners are there? 53
The impact of custody 54
The remand process 56
'Bailable' remand prisoners 58
Black defendants 59
Diversion from custody 59
Court assessment schemes 61
Diversion at the police custody stage 65
The inter-agency approach 66
What should be done? 67
Conclusion 69
References 70

5 **Recreating mayhem? Developing understanding for social
work with mentally disordered people** 72
MICHAEL PRESTON-SHOOT

Unravelling complexities, signposting interventions 72
Recreating mayhem? 73
Understanding and understandable practice 86
Conclusion 91
Cases 91
Circulars 91
References 91

**6   Multi-agency risk management of mentally disordered sex
offenders: a probation case study**   **95**

DANIEL GRANT

*Mental disorder and sex offending: some introductory
   considerations 95*
*The purpose and character of multi-agency intervention with
   mentally disordered sex offenders 96*
Rehabilitation and treatment revisited 98
Enhanced supervision 101
Sex Offender Risk Management Approach (SORMA) 102
Case study: Peter 103
Discussion 107
Conclusion 108
References 110

7   The Parole Board and the mentally disordered offender   **112**

JUDITH PITCHERS

Parole and risk: a new emphasis 112
Risk and the mentally disordered offender 114
The Parole Board's policy towards the mentally ill 116
Prisoners transferred to hospital 121
*Conclusion: risks to the public and risks to the rights of the
   mentally disordered 122*
References 125

**8   Control and compassion: the uncertain role of Mental
Health Review Tribunals in the management of the
mentally ill**   **127**

JOHN WOOD

Mental illness and legal restraint 127
The differing roles of psychiatry and law 128
The process of decision-making 130
The role of the tribunals re-examined 133
Conclusions 138
References 140

9 Thinking horses, not zebras 141

JILL PEAY

Inquiries after homicide 142
Actions for negligence 143
Effective communication and the human condition 145
Reasoning processes and responsibility 148
Clunis: wrecked or scuttled? 150
Acknowledgements 153
Notes 153
References 154

10 A balance of possibilities: some concluding notes on rights,
risks and the mentally disordered offender 156

DAVID WEBB

A test of the civilising process 158
Actuarial welfare and managing the mentally disordered
offender 161
Offender, deviant or patient? 165
Notes 166
References 166

Index 169

Contributors

Philip Bean is Professor of Criminology and Director of the Midlands Centre for Criminology and Criminal Justice at Loughborough University. He is the author or editor of eighteen books and many articles, mainly in the field of mental disorder. These include *Compulsory Admissions to Mental Hospitals* (John Wiley, 1980); *Mental Disorder and Legal Control* (Cambridge University Press, 1987) and (with Pat Mounser) *Discharged from Mental Hospitals* (Macmillan, 1994). In press is a book (for Macmillan) on mental disorder and social policy. From 1995 to 1999 Philip Bean was the President of the British Society of Criminology.

Sir Louis Blom-Cooper QC has had a distinguished career as a public law practitioner and in public administration. He was chairman of the Press Council (1989–90) and of the Mental Health Act Commission (1987–94), and has been the Independent Commissioner for the Holding Courts in Northern Ireland since 1993, charged with monitoring the regime of interviewing terrorist suspects in police custody. He has chaired numerous Panels of Inquiry, including those into the deaths of Jasmine Beckford (1985) and Kimberley Carlisle (1987); and in the mental health field, into the case of Jason Mitchell (1996) as well as into the allegations of ill-treatment of patients at Ashworth Hospital (1992) on which he comments in the present volume.

Paul Cavadino is Director of Policy and Information for the National Association for the Care and Resettlement of Offenders (NACRO). He is also Chair of the Penal Affairs Consortium, an alliance of thirty-five organisations concerned with the penal system, and clerk to the Parliamentary All-Party Penal Affairs Group. His recent publications include *An Introduction to the Criminal Justice Process* (Waterside Press, 1995) and *Children Who Kill* (Waterside Press, 1996).

Daniel Grant is a specialist practitioner in child protection. He developed the Sex Offender Risk Management Approach (SORMA) through investigative criminological research, for which he was awarded his PhD by the University of Hull. The practitioner emphasis of his work is increasingly concerned with multi-disciplinary training in methods of intervention with dangerous offenders.

Robert Harris is Professor in the Department of Politics and Asian Studies at the University of Hull, having formerly worked at Brunel and Leicester Universities (at the latter of which he was a junior colleague of Herschel Prins). He has a long-standing interest in criminology and criminal justice, and has published widely on juvenile justice, the probation service, secure accommodation and child care. He completed his work on this book during his tenure as Dorothy Lam Fellow at Hong Kong Baptist University.

Jill Peay is a Senior Lecturer in Law at the London School of Economics and an Associate Tenant at Doughty Street chambers. She is the author of *Tribunals on Trial: A Study of Decision-Making under the Mental Health Act 1983* (Clarendon Press, 1989) and *Enquiries After Homicide* (Duckworth, 1996) and *Criminal Justice and the Mentally Disordered* (Dartmouth, 1998).

Judith Pitchers was a member of the Parole Board for England and Wales from 1991 to 1997. She currently teaches at the Midlands Centre for Criminology and Criminal Justice at Loughborough University, and is a member of the Advisory Board on Restricted Patients. She has been a magistrate since 1979 and a member of the Board of Visitors at HMP Gartee since 1981. She is also a member of the Magisterial Committee of the Judicial Studies Board.

Michael Preston-Shoot is Professor of Social Work and Social Care at Liverpool John Moores University. He has written widely in the area of social work law and is currently involved in several projects on how community care law, policy and provision are experienced by service users and by practitioners.

David Webb is Head of the Department of Social Sciences and Dean of the Faculty of Economics and Social Science at Nottingham Trent University. He has in the past worked as a school teacher, an education adviser for the Central Council for Education and Training in Social Work and as a lecturer in sociology at Leicester University, where like Robert Harris he was a junior colleague of Herschel Prins.

Sir John Wood is Emeritus Professor in Law at the University of Sheffield, and is Chairman of the Trent Mental Health Review Tribunal.

Preface

This book is dedicated to Herschel Prins, who for a while in the late 1970s and early 1980s was the Director of the School of Social Work at the University of Leicester. We were then relatively junior lecturers, much given in those days to sometimes querulous interruptions to the intellectual and pedagogic life of the School, in the course of which we no doubt created a degree of irritation amongst our more established (but enduringly patient) colleagues.

Some of what we then – and later – wrote, stood as something of a debate with what we saw Herschel representing. But over time – and with increasing humility – we came to appreciate the moral and procedural complexities that were inherent in what Herschel was trying to convey when he was talking or writing about mentally disordered offenders. Running through his work are various distinctive themes: the tolerance of sometimes horrific behaviour alongside the moral imperative of loving the sinner whatever the sin; the need for professionals to work together with some humility, whatever might be the differences in the 'paradigms' they bring to the matter at hand; addressing honestly the risk posed by troublesome individuals and the importance of recognising that the public must be protected; speaking out against scapegoating the mentally disordered, and encouraging an informed debate about what a humane society ought to do to with (and for) some of its most challenging citizens. All these concerns resonate with what we thought – and still do think – is important in this particular corner of social welfare.

We have brought together a group of contributors who have in a variety of ways been influenced by the work of Herschel Prins. Despite being beyond retirement age he still works – with Visiting Professorships at the Department of Social Sciences at Nottingham Trent University and at the Midlands Centre for Criminology at Loughborough University – and two of the contributors (Philip Bean and Judith Pitchers) are current colleagues of his at Loughborough. Michael Preston-Shoot was a student at the School of Social Work in the 1970s, and has taken what he learnt from Herschel then into his current professorship in social work at John Moores University, Liverpool. Sir John Wood shared membership of the Mental Health Review Tribunal, as well as having a common academic interest in mentally disordered offenders. Daniel Grant is a doctoral student with

Robert Harris at Hull, and, guided by his supervisor, has drawn on Herschel Prins' work for his research into the treatment regimes for sex offenders. Jill Peay is herself an expert on the socio-legal aspects of mentally disordered offending, so her connection is the collegial one of 'the academy', whilst the contribution from Paul Cavadino of NACRO is an expression of the impact that Herschel has had on the world of criminal justice policy and practice.

Our own contributions reflect an involvement in this area that is less to do with the specific field of mental disorder, than with the commonalities between this and some general themes within social welfare, criminal justice and criminology. In part, this reflects the particular division of labour within the academy, but it is also a demonstration in line with what one of our contributors – Jill Peay – has elsewhere argued, namely that mentally disordered offenders should not be treated as an isolated category (Peay, 1994: 1154), but that the issues they pose ought to be seen as part of a more generic set of social welfare considerations.

Nevertheless, there is a distinctive and substantive solidity of writing and teaching in the field of the mentally disordered offender to which Herschel Prins has added considerably, and it is this which is, in a way, the point of departure for this collection. Over more than thirty years he has established himself with an imposing contribution to a wider understanding of people who are often amongst our most troubled (and, it has to be said, most troublesome) citizens. Those who have benefited from Herschel Prins' thoughtful and insightful scholarship include lawyers, psychiatrists. social workers and probation officers, although the clearly written and refreshingly accessible nature of his books and articles has extended this to a readership well beyond those with an exclusively professional interest in the subject.

The humanising and civilising impact of Herschel Prins' approach to how we think about (or in professional guise 'assess') and respond to (or 'treat' or 'manage') mentally disordered offenders has been both impressive and influential. But his work never overlooks the 'reality' that mentally disordered people often have a dislocating (and frequently distressing) impact on their fellow citizens. Accordingly, this collection echoes the concerns to which Herschel Prins has himself returned repeatedly – that 'management' should be above all a benign instrument of what can be called (accurately, if a trifle ponderously) medico-juridical-welfare intervention. Reflecting to some extent such a tripartite arrangement, this collection touches – if sometimes obliquely – on the domains of *medicine* (as the 'scientific' attempt to understand the mind that is 'distorted'), the *law* (as offering guidance to citizens as to rights and duties as well as stipulating the relationship between punishment and capacity to conform), and *probation and social work* (as the expression of what has been called 'altruism under social auspices').

In marking – slightly belatedly, it has to be admitted – Herschel Prins' seventieth year, we hope that this collection points to the continuity between the work that he has himself undertaken on managing the mentally disordered offender, and that of others who have been influenced by his writing. We later say that this subject provides a test of how far a society has progressed in the civilising process, as it struggles to cope with sometimes frightening or bizarre behaviour whilst simultaneously resisting the retributive impulse. Herschel Prins has surely contributed to prompting and prodding our thinking along in the right direction, and this *Festschrift* is one attempt to mark the measure of that impact.

David Webb
Robert Harris
September1998

Reference

Peay, J. (1994) 'Mentally disordered offenders'. In M. Maguire, R. Morgan and R. Reines (eds) *The Oxford Handbook of Criminology*. Oxford: Clarendon Press.

Introduction

David Webb and Robert Harris

When considering the art of assembling an edited book, there seemed to us two options open to those bringing a collection of potentially disparate pieces together so far as an introduction is concerned. One – which reflects a robust insistence on self-improvement and an impatience with fashionable spoon-feeding – is to offer the various contributions without commentary, the reader being expected to get on with it and make their own sense of matters. The other – more self-consciously pedagogical and under the sway of the contemporary inclination to offer consumer guidance on everything – assumes that the responsibility of editing extends to offering a summary of all that follows, a kind of Reader's Digest that obviates the need for independent struggle with sometimes complex ideas. We equivocate in these matters. It has to be admitted that seventeen years or so of neo-liberalism undoubtedly leaves its mark, and there remains a legacy of irritation at feeling you are doing the work that others should do. On the other hand, there is perhaps a rather stronger residue of another sort of puritanism, one which invites an obligation to the reader who had parted with money or time to consider the contents of something which, whilst of indisputable worth in its own right, is also some sort of commodity. In marking the necessary exchanges that take place in these transactions, we eventually considered that discharging obligations through a summarising introduction was most fitting. However, and consistent with the spirit on these new times in which we now live, we have balanced our authorial duty with an expectation that the reader will assume personal responsibility for interpreting what follows in the body of the book. In other words, we have left enough unsaid to ensure that things are not made too easy.

The introductory chapter – by Robert Harris – is deliberately wide-ranging, designed as it is to set within a general framework of welfare and criminological concerns the specific instance of the mentally disordered offender. Harris talks of what he calls the 'outlier' status of mentally disordered offenders, caught as they are within the interstices of numerous agencies of control and regulation. This reflects the territory that Herschel Prins has covered in his own work in trying to unpack not only the complexities of the phenomenon, in both its aetiology as well as in the most appropriate way to manage the mentally disturbed offender. These people present as being categorically awkward, since they are neither exclusively 'ill', nor as uncomplicatedly 'bad'. The policy and practice responses accordingly totter between two not always compatible discourses of state intervention – in essence, when to medically treat an illness and when to penalise a legal infraction. And often we get this hopelessly wrong, reflecting all manner of cultural and penological muddle-headedness: these might be people who have done dreadful things, who although patently mad we still have an inclination to punish. The spiral of control intensifies in consequence. Even those whose waywardness is minor and who are kept out of prison find that the far from tender mercies of 'community care' do little to address their needs for treatment and support as mentally disturbed citizens. The nub of the matter – not surprisingly – is what we should do about those criminals who have varying degrees of reason at their command. The conclusion reached by Robert Harris is that if we do not do this very well, then we need to look at how we reconcile what is often only a rhetorical adherence to civilised care for the unfortunate, with a cultural force that expresses another of modernity's inclinations, namely that of preserving public order against the actually or potentially disruptive in our midst.

A key characteristic of modernity is the necessity of establishing 'the facts' in situations where something has gone wrong, and taking rational and systematic steps to rectify the situation. Another dimension of this clash between madness and rationality to which Harris refers lies in the fact that not only are mentally disordered offenders themselves liable to behave in disturbing or confusing ways, but this behaviour can in turn provoke behaviour no less outrageous (indeed one can plausibly argue much more so because it is less excusable) in those charged with the always difficult and often poorly rewarded job of caring for them; sometimes with tragic consequences.

Sir Louis Blom-Cooper QC and Herschel Prins have both chaired committees of inquiry into things that have gone wrong in mental hospitals, particularly the Special Hospitals where the most difficult and dangerous cases reside, as well as in the functioning of community care. They have done so from different premises and, therefore, in different ways. Blom-Cooper takes as the axis of his chapter the contrasting approaches taken by two committees of inquiry, one chaired by Herschel Prins and one by himself, which addressed somewhat similar issues in different Special Hospitals at about the same time. From this contrast he argues that inquiries, which are set up to allay public disquiet, should normally take place in public, with legal services available to those who wish them, so challenging Prins's view that a more informal and private approach is better suited to securing the confidence of those involved, and extracting from them their often complex and multifaceted interpretations of events.

Where the truth lies in such an argument is for readers to judge, though in doing so they will doubtless remember that in this chapter they have only one side of the case. Perhaps, however, the difference between Prins and Blom-Cooper is explained not only by different interpretations of empirical data about alternative modes of inquiry (for such data would, to put it mildly, be hard to come across in valid or reliable form). Of equal relevance may be the different models of mankind espoused by optimistic social worker and sceptical lawyer. The former's stock in trade is the avoidance of judgmentalism, drawing out the reluctant interviewee by creating a 'safe' environment in which complex, subtle and sensitive issues can be aired by people of goodwill who have, presumably, done their best in a difficult situation. The lawyer, however, is more likely to incline to the view that when it comes down to it, those with something to hide will seldom come clean unless pressed, that the public will be rightly sceptical of justice which is not seen to be done, and that only by exposing all testimony to public scrutiny by the legal representatives of the parties involved – some of whom will certainly be insufficiently astute or articulate to conduct the proceedings on their own behalf – can the danger of injustice or professional cover-up be minimised.

If this interpretation of a significant difference of view between an eminent social worker and an eminent lawyer whose mutual respect is beyond question is correct, it highlights once again the difficulty involved in securing the inter-professional collaboration which everybody believes crucial if work with mentally disordered offenders is to be done in a comprehensive and coherent way: with the best will in the world, different professions just see things differently.

While, on the one hand, there is arguably cause to celebrate this diversity of perspective, on the other, this kind of argument is perhaps best held in the context of training and not 'live cases'. The fundamental nature of the difference of view highlights just how far we are from giving effect to a true multi-disciplinarity which, perhaps, will be achieved only when the various disciplines undergo joint pre-professional training, and do so in an academically as well as professionally oriented institution, where these cultural differences can be argued out in an open and non-defensive way.

This theme of the problematic nature of multi-disciplinarity surfaces repeatedly in this book. For example, in his contribution, Philip Bean discusses the way in which the police – and police surgeons in particular – play a key role in dealing with the mentally disordered in a public place. Given the absence of alternatives, the police station more often than not becomes the place of safety to which a mentally disordered person is removed, and this fact sets the mould for the criminalisation of something that was initially not intended to be a criminal matter. The decarceration movement – and its policy expression in Community Care – has exacerbated this tendency for the police station to be the point where the mentally disordered person is sucked into the criminal justice system rather than the health care one. This is in part because of the sheer difficulty in establishing other sites as places of safety: Bean is especially critical of the problems that face the police in securing cooperation from the medical and nursing professions in using hospitals for this purpose. But equally he says that the tendency of the police to rely on police surgeons, described by him as 'these apparently unimportant figures, almost wholly neglected in the research literature, [who] may well turn out to be the key', contributes to the problem. The failure to call upon an Approved Social Worker, and the reliance on perfunctory and superficial assessments by a police surgeon are viewed by Bean as part of that process which sees too many mentally disordered offenders routed inappropriately into the penal system.

Bean points up one mechanism of 'net widening', as local decision-making and unhelpful inter-professional cooperation expand the coercive social control to which vulnerable people are subject. In his chapter, Paul Cavadino is also concerned with the way in which 'disposals' (a generic and rather Benthamite word, but one which nevertheless conveys something that could be imprisonment, community service, or explicitly medical treatment) might best meet the particular needs of those who are mentally disordered. He points to a number of demonstration projects that have brought professionals together to successfully divert offenders who are mentally disordered from prison. By calling on the appropriate psychiatric and social work expertise at the point of being initially apprehended by the police, the scope to route the individual through the health care system is that much greater. Nevertheless it is important to recognise – as Cavadino emphasises – that diversion without support is worthless; it requires health care support that is appropriately matched to the psychiatric and social needs of these people. But at the same time, it has to be recognised that the fact of being mentally disordered is not on its own sufficient to warrant diversion. Issues to do with dangerousness and public protection have to be considered, though the woefully inadequate provision of psychiatric provision does not enjoin courts to have consideration of health care in prison hospitals. The fact that prisoners have no right of access to the NHS raises further questions (ethical as well as medical) about the potentially destructive consequences of imprisonment for those who are mentally disordered.

Cavadino conveys something of a system that often latches onto a particular disposal because no one has any idea what else to do. Remands for psychiatric and social reasons can see mentally disordered offenders in prison because 'something needs to be done' for people who are patently troubled, so that proportionality and risk are set aside in pursuit of hopelessly misplaced benevolence. The fact that the Bail Act does not require courts to have consideration of the implications of the mental condition of the accused when considering an application for bail adds to the spiral of expanded sanctioning of those who are mentally disturbed.

The consequences of diversion from imprisonment sees the invocation of other discourses, and one of these is social work, which plays an important part in holding the ring so far as community support is concerned. Michael Preston-Shoot sets this particular professional mandate within a range of impediments, ranging from resource shortages for the proper delivery of services, to the fact of having to work with extremely troubled people and the inter-personal (and intra-personal) psychodynamics that arise from this. Indeed, it is more than likely that the 'unwanted feelings and anxieties' which are generated by mentally disordered people account for the sometime indifference towards the distribution of resources to support them. But either way, the accumulated consequences of all this amplify the excluded and 'outlier' status of the mentally disturbed, whatever 'pure' ethical imperatives might be claimed for the underpinning value base of social work. Given the complex and demanding nature of these 'cases', and the high visibility that arises when things are seen to go wrong, it is not surprising that social work agencies look to the bureaucratisation of procedures in order to allay organisational anxiety. Individual workers, unless supported imaginatively, will be inclined the same way. The recourse to excessive legalism is something which Preston-Shoot regards with concern, diverting as it does social work from its mission to work within those very interstices about which Robert Harris lays such conceptual emphasis.

In large measure, the way out for Michael Preston-Shoot is the realignment of the values upon which social work with mentally disturbed offenders rests; as he says, 'values are central to preventing professional and organisational abuse of individuals', though he stresses that this is not simply a matter of holding these by individual workers (which would be idealistic in both the popular and technical sense of the term), but that these values should be embedded in, and expressed through, policy and organisational structures. Through this, some of the evident failings that emerge in the way in which we manage the mentally disordered offender through community care might be alleviated, lifting the disavowal to which they are subjected. Echoing the emphasis that Herschel Prins makes about the importance at least of 'naming' the dynamics of working with the sometimes difficult, the sometimes unlovable and the sometimes unpleasant, Michael Preston-Shoot argues for an ethical base that guards against the wilder excesses of some baser instincts.

Part of the impediment to delivering community-based support for mentally disturbed offenders surrounds the seemingly intractable problems of multi-agency working, though it is true that in his chapter, Paul Cavadino does point to some notable successes in collaboration to ensure diversion from custody. But once diverted, what is to happen? Daniel Grant provides an account of multi-agency cooperation operating under the coordinating auspices of the probation service. The vehicle for this is the telling instance of a case study, in which several agencies come together to meet those who simultaneously present challenges that routinely characterise this field – namely supporting the health needs of someone who is mentally disturbed and commits 'trivial' misdemeanours, but who at the same time poses what could be a *potential* danger to the community greater than would be suggested from the nature of those offences. Here be those troubled waters of dangerousness, prediction, community safety, respect for the person and sheer blind professional panic.

Sex offending is a particular test of professional and organisational resolve, for reasons so obvious that they need not be spelled out here. But if this can be controlled – and Grant takes the stance of pragmatic restraint, rather than the chimera of 'treatment' as his objective – then this offers another form of effective community-based management in which diversion and risk-minimising public protection can both be met. Of course, this places probation within a paradigm that is explicitly control-oriented and this is certainly not without its critics, as Grant reminds us. But he also maintains that in so far as control reduces recidivism then the path to rehabilitation is made easier and this is surely important. It is for this reason that 'enhanced supervision' is a legitimate method for the probation service to adopt. It depends crucially on a measure of seamlessness in the operation of the various agencies concerned with an offender, in which high-level surveillance and the sharing of intelligence about behaviour are employed to ensure that risk is contained. Grant spells out the constituent elements of the Sex Offender Risk Management Approach (SORMA) that he has developed, in which explicit control, situational crime prevention, the exercise of legislative authority and multi-agency collaboration are amongst the underpinning principles for this particular form of management. SORMA blends the new pragmatism of 'what works' probation practice with aspects of realist criminology and the kind of actuarial welfare that lays considerable emphasis on detailed risk assessment. The case study that Grant introduces illustrates these principles operating in practice, showing how high-level surveillance and the exchange of intelligence on offender behaviour offer something that aims for the scrutiny afforded by the Panopticon combined with the spatial relaxation of decarceration. The outcome in this particular case could in one sense be seen as a 'failure', but this is to miss the point. Even if what in the USA is sometimes called 'incapacitation' (the legal disqualification of various freedoms, most notably liberty) is the eventual result of community intervention, the important thing to have established is a secure moral basis for that detention – as it is to have tried as hard as possible to prevent the withdrawal of liberty happening in the first place. And as is said from time to time in this book, the management of mentally disordered offenders indeed demands an acknowledgement that sometimes incapacitation is entirely appropriate.

Nevertheless, there should be restraints on the power of the state to incarcerate, and this might be particularly so when detention is somehow linked with the exercise of professional judgement over the clinical state of a mentally disordered person. The Parole Board is part of the institution of checks and balances that a modern state adopts to demonstrate that there is some limit to what is always in danger of being seen as its arbitrariness. The Parole Board thereby contributes to the legitimation of power so that it can be used with authority. Judith Pitchers' contribution explores the way in which the Parole Board is part of the risk assessment culture of deviancy management. The basis for deciding whether or not to grant parole seems eminently reasonable – good behaviour whilst in prison together with a favourable prognosis about future waywardness ought to have its own rewards. But risk, however slight it might be, always entails the possibility that something untoward may happen, though as she argues, *in general* the Parole Board seems to select prisoners for parole whose risk of offending is lower than average.

The situation is not so rosy for mentally disordered offenders, who are seen by the Board as posing risks so high that the frequency of parole being granted for them is very low. Judith Pitchers offers an inferential account of what might be happening so far as mentally disordered offenders are concerned. She casts doubt on the adequacy of the risk assessments that are provided to the Board, noting, along with others contributing to this volume, that this is a notoriously imprecise area of forensic activity anyway. She suggests too that release plans provided by the probation service are often insufficiently robust to make the Board confident about supervision in the community – which makes the model developed by Grant that much more significant. In general, it seems that the information available to the Board means that it is unable to differentiate adequately between those offenders who pose serious threats to the community and those who do not, and in order to avoid the impact on public confidence from being seen to have got it wrong, the tendency is to adopt a rule of pessimism and 'play safe'. Judith Pitchers concludes that of course the Board has to have due regard to the community and its protection, but this ought not be at the expense of injustice towards the mentally disturbed offender.

This balance between competing objectives and ethical imperatives is given particular explicitness in the chapter by John Wood, which is concerned with the right to a periodic challenge to the State's incapacitation of those who are mentally disturbed. The Mental Health Review Tribunals – like the Parole Board – exist to demonstrate that the State is not indeed Leviathan. He argues that there are two 'contradictory forces' at work in the administration of detaining those who have a mental disorder: a paternalistic concern for those who are ill, about whom the experts have the voice, and the advancement of personal liberties that are enshrined in common law. In arbitrating this, tribunals serve as the forum to review the case of those who have been compulsorily hospitalised under the Mental Health Act 1983, presenting an opportunity for the patient to present arguments for the discharging of the Order. The structure of the tribunal, on the face of it at least, is quasi-judicial, with the case for continued incapacitation being set against that of release. In essence this leads to a dialogue between the discourses of medicine and law, with lawyers seeking to test the robustness of the case made by psychiatrists. Although this could collapse into adversarialism, John Wood considers that this is not what usually happens, with Tribunals seeking, in investigative fashion, to weigh up the evidence from a variety of quarters and reaching a considered conclusion accordingly.

This describes what happens in terms of formal procedures, though there is another 'reading' of matters to which we are guided, and this concerns the latent function – or the symbolism – of the events surrounding tribunals. John Wood is himself quite explicit about this, confessing to 'an unease about the true purpose of the Mental Health Review Tribunal system'. He notes that 'the proportion of patients whose Order is discharged is so small as to give the impression that the exercise itself is misconceived', but goes on to articulate a view which talks of the importance of the hearing as a means by which worries and concerns that are held by the patient, or by those who are in some way their advocates, might be brought to the attention of the hospital authorities. Less a juridical exercise in the exercise of rights, tribunals act administratively as a conduit of representation and more effective case management. This is clearly John Wood's preference. The approach avoids the undue formality of a court and retains a sense of serving the patient, and at the same time it indicates to the world at large that there exists ways in which periodic review of detention demonstrates the reasonableness of the State's actions to incapacitate in the first place. This might create the impression of a certain 'constitutional fuzziness', recalling Robert Harris's point about mental health operating within a multitude of interstices and with an absence of 'proper' arrangements in place to deal with some very difficult issues. Certainly, seen in this light the disjuncture between the formal and the latent functions of Mental Health Review Tribunals presents an interesting perspective on the management of disorder.

A caution towards the formality of legal processes is also of thematic significance in Jill Peay's chapter, where the implications of the 'inquiry industry' busily investigating the committing of homicide by mentally disordered offenders is examined. Above all, these inquiries have begun to generate a climate within which the retrospective ascription of culpability for negligence has begun to have an impact on the delivery of services to mentally disordered offenders. Inquiries build up a certain sort of picture, which in the vernacular would say that there is nothing as sure as 20:20 hindsight, or as Peay herself puts it more circumspectly, 'hindsight tends to produce inflated perceptions of foreseeability and of the relevance of data preceding an event'. The cumulative narrative that is built up from inquiries as they retrospectively re-order 'the facts', is essentially one that suggests that everything was obvious from the outset and that anyone who missed the startlingly obvious must be incompetent, negligent or indolent. One consequence of this is that an accumulation of evidence from inquiries might lead authorities to create ever more complex guidelines within which their staff must operate, yet which might have the unintended consequence of strangulating the creative management of mental disorder that depends – as Grant shows – on the fluidity of operating across professional boundaries and the willingness to be guided by the inferential and sometimes by the intuitive.

This reminds us that matters are – as ever with this topic – frighteningly messy. The manifold difficulties in approaching the subject of managing the mentally disordered offender that have engaged Herschel Prins for so long are returned to in the final chapter by David Webb. Balancing the protection of the community with the rights of individuals about whom we might have the gravest concern and suspicions is not easy. The problems in predicting dangerousness and the impossibility of giving a level of assurance about the degree of risk that the community might feel it deserves are endemic themes in this area, as are the decisions that have to be taken about the extent to which we are prepared to vary the principles of accountability in the case of those whose reasonableness is less than that of others – always assuming that there is a datum of reasonableness that can be used to fix the mind of the wayward. The enduringly flawed way in which we resolve – or, rather, fail to resolve – the assigning of mentally disordered offenders to the domains either of health or of penality, is a measure of wider confusions in the cognitive map that we hold of citizens whom we are unsure whether to blame or to pity. As with the work of Herschel Prins, this seems an appropriate thing to worry away at, and it is something that all the following contributions do in their varying ways.

Chapter 1

Mental disorder and social order

Underlying themes in crime management

Robert Harris[1]

> Thus psychiatric knowledge, then in full spate of development, was introduced in this indirect fashion into the enforcement of the law . . . The criminal lunatic, as harmful, if not more harmful to the social order than any other criminal, had to be condemned, but his status as madman took precedence over his status as criminal. Any and all experts on the facts concerned were as qualified as the judges to determine responsibility by the primacy conferred on the facts of a case and the context of the offender's behavior over the offense itself . . . The result, therefore, is to diminish the specific character of law enforcement and to reduce the power of the judges, since their specific jurisdiction is invaded by experts of various kinds.
>
> (Moulin 1975: 215)

The subject matter of this book is not, as our contributors make plain, and as the work of Herschel Prins, whose work we look to honour in this *Festschrift*, amply demonstrates, straightforward. To the present author, steeped for many years in criminology, social and political theory and policy-oriented criminal justice, but addressing the problems posed by mentally disordered offenders for the first time, not only do a number of logical and conceptual conundrums surface and invite consideration, but the act of considering them teaches us much about mainstream concerns in criminology. Looking at how we comprehend the seemingly irrational few tells us how we comprehend, without even thinking about them, the taken-for-granted seemingly rational many. This chapter, then, is written by an outsider to the sub-discipline of mentally disordered offenders who, in the outsider's time-honoured role, seeks to expose some of these conundrums to a scrutiny only minimally infected by the normal assumptions of the experts.

For all the vagaries of politics and economics which drive particular micro-policies (such as the application by health, local authorities, police and others of the *minutiae* of legislation – see, for example, Bean's chapter in the present volume) or *mezzo*-policies (such as the replacement of mental hospitals with a set of aspirations euphemistically termed 'community care' but more accurately designated 'pass the parcel'), the ways in which we manage mentally disordered offenders are expressions of culturally located perceptions of madness and crime.

Accordingly, this chapter raises issues, in particular those surrounding the place of 'reason' in the management of crime, which daily confront those who deal with, and struggle to comprehend, the management of mentally disordered offenders.

Herschel Prins falls into both these camps, and his achievements, as scholar, teacher, consultant and long-serving member of a mental health review tribunal, are widely recognised. Prins has never fought shy of engaging with the most insoluble of social problems, drawing frequently on artistic insights into human personality and behaviour (see, for example, Prins 1995: Chapter 10). For Prins, to understand the totality of these phenomena we must examine not only the objects of therapeutic attention but those who administer the therapy. They, far from being clinical automata, have, like everybody else, feelings, beliefs and attitudes which, while they may help or hinder their work, can scarcely avoid affecting it. Prins therefore challenges professionals to address and interpret those parts of their personality and behaviour which others might consider off court; to Herschel Prins, professionals who would manage mentally disordered offenders should first show they can manage themselves.

This, then, is not a chapter which offers many solutions, but by addressing some of the more interesting issues to surface about mental disorder and crime, it exposes for consideration solutions which already exist – or which are purported to exist. They may or may not be good solutions; certainly, they are not invariably articulated by professionals or politicians, but because they feature in the explanations discussed by other contributors, they are worth consideration at this early point in our book.

Mental disorder and criminality: some boundary issues

> we are all brought up to believe that we may inflict injuries on anyone against whom we can make out a case of moral inferiority.
>
> (George Bernard Shaw 1941: 13)

Mentally disordered offenders bear two characteristics which sit in uneasy relation to each other. Clearly it is possible to be classified mentally disordered but not be an offender. Equally, in both workaday politics and professional beliefs, calculative and behavioural theories have largely superseded those psycho-pathological explanations which once led some to conclude that the commission of a deviant act was itself sufficient evidence of mental difficulty for some clinical remedy to be worthy of consideration. Accordingly, one can now be an offender without too much risk of one's criminal behaviour being exposed to psychological or psychiatric scrutiny.

When, however, we encounter someone who is by common consent both mentally disordered and a criminal it is difficult though necessary to determine the relation between the two conditions (see, for example, Feldman 1977: 162–165; Moir and Jessel 1995: Chapter 13). This problem exists in part because of the requirement of the M'Naghten Test that the onus be placed on the defence to demonstrate a causal link between a disease of the mind and the crime committed (Feldman 1977: 162). It is also implicitly acknowledged in the softening of the then extant insanity defence, by the introduction of the notion of 'diminished responsibility' (for practical purposes by the Homicide Act 1957, though for an indication of earlier legislation, see Gunn 1991: 21). The more hesitant ethos of this phrase creates a calibrated notion of responsibility which transforms insanity from an absolute into a relative concept. Though translating these calibrations into law and policy has proved difficult in the extreme, the concept had its practical manifestation in the reforms heralded by the Mental Health Acts 1959 and, in the light of the recommendations of the Butler Committee (Home Office and Department of Health and Social Security 1975), 1983.[2]

How we measure these relativities is in good part a forensic problem. We might in practice take the view that, irrespective of law, the crimes of the mentally disordered are, except in a very few cases, satisfactorily explained by the mental disorder from which the criminal is suffering. This clinical judgement is, however, in the hands of forensic psychiatrists and other professionals whose diagnostic and predictive expertise has not emerged unscathed from critical scrutiny (for contrasting perspectives, see Glueck 1963; Gerber 1984) and whose clinical judgements appear heavily influenced by subjective preference. So, in the view of an academic psychologist, discussing the trial of the mass murderer Sutcliffe, whom a jury declared sane but who was transferred to a special hospital three years after conviction:

> It is rather hard to resist the view that, in the cold light of day, it is faintly ludicrous to have to debate at great length the normality of an individual who *behaves* toward other people in the way which Sutcliffe did.
>
> (Hollin 1989: 125)

On the other hand, according to a senior judge: 'Only infrequently will the factors that make a man mad also operate directly to make him offend' (Mustill 1991: 225–226). That there are profound tactical consequences of either of these views is self-evident. If virtually any crime committed by the mentally disordered involved exoneration through insanity or alleviation of guilt through diminished responsibility, the socio-political choice would be between giving the offender a blank cheque to offend and making a response geared not to the traditional purposes of justice or punishment (which can scarcely be appropriate if volition is denied) but to public protection, with a consequential elevation of security over rights. If forensic psychiatry and related professional discourses are indeed as subjective as this (Floud and Young 1981: *passim*, but in particular Appendix C; Craft and Craft 1984: *passim*), the idea that fine distinctions can be reliably drawn between the rational and the irrational, with precise degrees of responsibility ascribed to some configuration of person, incident, time and place, appears a little optimistic.

If the diagnostic problems which arise with those who occupy the disputed territory between the clinical and the penal confront professionals and intellectuals with the empirical as well as conceptual inadequacy of their own dichotomies, then the question of disposal presents a similar problem. There is no clear concept in Western culture of anything 'between' a hospital and a prison (Harris and Timms 1993).[3] Accordingly, the problem, in a curative environment such as a hospital, of conceptualising the management of someone for whom cure is unlikely but who should not, through lack of volition in his or her criminality, go to prison either, is acute. The fact that both nomenclature and funding arrangements differ between 'hospitals' for mentally disordered serious offenders and 'prisons' for their mentally ordered counterparts may be a source of greater satisfaction to intellectuals and policy-makers than to the criminals themselves, for whom the experience of incarceration is presumably much the same whichever Department of State provides the facility. Indeed, the claim that the hospitals in which they are being held are doing anything other than the job of a prison might even appear to them a little casuistic. At the same time though, few informed people wish prisons to be overtly punitive, and even if they do, the existence of international standards (for example, United Nations 1988) and the activities of the Council of Europe make such an approach inconceivable in the United Kingdom.

So mentally disordered offenders present problems of organisational responsibility, falling as they do within the interlocking areas of health, social services, probation and prison. They are seldom viewed by exponents of any of these disciplines as especially promising material; their clinical conditions characteristically lack precise diagnosis (Blackburn 1993) and where such a diagnosis exists, it is liable to be couched in terms which leave only minimal room for curative optimism. Seemingly through combined limitations of resource and imagination, they make demands on the system and those who work in it of a kind which cannot easily be met (Mace 1991; Pinder and Laming 1991). To professions which operate in a political and cultural context in which solution finding is critical for professional status, they are, as the most hopeless of cases, doomed to marginalisation unless they become such a nuisance as to render themselves eligible for therapeutic or penal coercion.

While some mentally disordered offenders may lead professionals to believe that they will in the future fall into this 'nuisance' category, relatively few actually do – many fewer than psychiatrists often predict (Craft 1984; Prins 1986: 87–89). Accordingly, given the closures of mental hospitals and the refusal of successive governments to replace them with an effective community care system, individuals of minor disorder and minor criminality who are not sent to prison (as they should not be, according to activists: see Staite *et al.* 1994; Cavadino, this volume) are expected to live in what can only in the loosest sense be described as the community – 'community' usually meaning, in this context, 'not in an institution'.

Order, disorder and all stations in between

> the recognition of biological and sociocultural causality in human behavior
> does not exclude altogether a realistic concept of capacity for choice which
> different persons possess in varying degree.
>
> (Glueck 1963: 15)

The mentally disordered offender is a borderline figure – between mental disorder and criminality, criminality and social problem, petty nuisance and social casualty – and thus presents a serious categorical problem for both judicial and social policy. Neo-classical justice systems can only operate with popular consent if procedures exist for the recategorisation of those outliers for whom the imposition of a tariff sentence would be widely perceived as inappropriate or unjust. It follows that outliers have to be dealt with differently from routine cases, if only to sustain confidence that the system as a whole is just and reasonable to the 'common man'. This stricture applies to other groups, including children and, sometimes, women (for a useful review, see Heidensohn 1994), who are processed within a criminal justice system geared mainly to the efficient disposal of the able-bodied, able-minded adult male offenders who constitute the bulk of its objects.

Mentally disordered offenders are a further example of such an outlier,[4] but for judicial disposal, even assuming we can agree who is in and not in this category, many of them are not so much taxonomically distinct (and distinctive) as hard cases who make bad law. Accordingly, a perceived absence of reason on the part of an offender provokes equivocation among judicial administrators, policy-makers and practitioners, to the last of whom it falls to choose between the paradigms of 'madness' and 'badness' in the process of selecting an appropriate disposal. Even today, pure reason, though doubtless never encountered, is vaunted in popular culture as the proper basis for social, economic and political relations almost as much as it was in the Enlightenment. It follows that if a category of people exists who cannot be expected to respond rationally to punishment, persuading them to conform to legally and socially sanctioned expectations becomes awkward. This awkwardness stems from the precise logical problem that our predominant means of persuasion, being reason-based, is dependent for its success on the similar existence of reason in the objects of our persuasive endeavours. How can reason persuade the unreasoned in the absence of a common language, a convincing rhetoric, by which to engage with them? Yet because the objects of this persuasion, though deficient in reason, lack nothing in nuisance value, action of some kind must assuredly be taken.

Considerations such as this have led some scholars to dispute the wisdom of any kind of insanity defence, including its contemporary descendant diminished responsibility (for relevant discussions, see Radzinowicz and Turner 1944; Feldman 1977; Grounds 1991; Blackburn 1993). Others have reached a somewhat similar conclusion by a different route. Gostin, for example, takes the view that therapeutic care is but a thinly veiled and inadequately accountable mode of coercion:

If one examines the insanity defence carefully, it becomes clear that its purpose is not to absolve mentally ill people from penal consequences but rather to authorise confinement in cases where the law would not ordinarily allow such confinement.

(Gostin 1984: 228)

This being so, says Gostin, let the mentally disordered have their disorder looked after, but keep this separate from their criminality, which should be dealt with no more coercively than would have occurred had the offender not been deemed disordered. In other words, forget metaphysical concepts such as 'insanity' or 'motive', and sentence at the level warranted by the crime, independently of questions about responsibility.

It is hard not to feel that the attractiveness of such an approach to Gostin and civil libertarians like him is dependent in good part on the empirical accuracy of the claim that the law works to the disadvantage of mentally disordered offenders. But even setting aside the fact that in some cases mental disorder mitigates the harshness of sentence (Gostin's proposal accordingly condemning those mentally disordered offenders who excite judicial sympathy to additional harshness), the idea that mentally disordered offenders should be sentenced as though they were sane, but treated as though they were not, would seem hard to defend.

Studying a marginal case like mentally disordered offenders confronts us with the reality that the boundaries between sanity and insanity, rationality and irrationality, crime and disease, social nuisance and social casualty, prison and hospital, even offender and therapist, become increasingly blurred the more one questions the robustness of the categorisations themselves. Herschel Prins, as we have seen, is interested in the richness and complexity of human personality and behaviour, and in the aesthetic sensibility of professionals as well as offenders. To Prins, in the world of human relations, rationality and dispassion are seldom achieved and not always achievable, and a more intuitive empathy is required, albeit an empathy to be harnessed in the service of the traditional characteristics of professionalism, such as consistency of treatment and quality of service.

In adhering to this approach, Prins gets close to one of the paradoxes of his field. For if trained experts cannot be relied upon to act like experimental scientists, but share some of the irrationality, impulsiveness, fears and fantasies of their charges, how can we posit the existence of a binary divide between sanity and madness, mental order and mental disorder? If in the faces of their clients or patients the professionals see, as it were, their own brother or sister if not themselves, how can they talk calmly of objectivity or detachment? To make a point which characterises many human service professions working with many client groups, how can they unyoke the therapy from the therapist? Or, in Yeats's words, 'tell the dancer from the dance'?

This question has been debated from a number of perspectives. Philosophically, once we move away from the notion that pure reason exists, decontextualised from time and place, (see, for example, Norrie 1986), or that any choice can be wholly free (see, for example, Blackburn 1993), the idea of a dichotomy between mental disorder and mental order begins to fragment. But if none of us is an exemplification of pure reason, the understanding of disorder itself becomes as central to our concerns as the relation between such disorder and criminality. As we have seen, the concept 'diminishment' has gone some way towards deconstructing this dualism, but at the point of application, the courts are still faced with a binary opposition between diminishment and non-diminishment; and it is at least as much at the point of application as at that of conceptualisation that problems of managing the mentally disordered offender occur.

So from the literature surveyed one concludes that the classification of mental disorder is itself unsound (the word 'subjective' appears repeatedly). It is seen by some as a moral categorisation and by others as a justification for a form and degree of social control not justifiable under laws framed for the disposal of 'sane' criminals; while others, on the contrary, see the question of individual mental disorder as largely irrelevant, since the fundamental purpose of the legal system is the removal of social disorder and the creation of social order based on collective reason. In this rather utilitarian approach, it is social order which constitutes the socio-political bedrock of a civilised society. That the same word defines a desirable individual mental state and a desirable social state simply signifies that social order can only be secured by the removal of disordered (and so irrational and unpredictable) elements. As madness and crime are by definition aspects of disorder, the disordered state of individuals becomes, independently of volition, as much a potential contributor to social disorder as crime, therefore demanding equally firm management.

Accordingly, in this argument the only difference between the treatment of the 'sane' and the 'insane' is the carceral mechanism deployed; hence emerges what has been termed the paradox of: 'calls for diverting the mentally disordered offender from the damaging effects of the criminal justice system . . . yet, on the other hand, concerns remain about some discharged mental patients and the likelihood of their reoffending' (Peay 1994: 1120). Taking as their starting point that the justice system is – though heavily secularised today – based on outmoded theological notions of individual rationality, proponents of the primacy of order thesis argue that the system drives us to a position in which those deemed mentally *disordered* are handled in a categorically different way from those implicitly deemed (and only implicitly, for, being 'normal' they do not need to be deemed anything at all) mentally *ordered*. According to this thesis, since mentally ordered offenders have reason they are to be punished because they have set aside goodness and, knowingly and deliberately, taken the *via sinistra*. Mentally disordered offenders, on the other hand, lack the rationality which permits the choice of good or evil, and therefore should not be punished, but treated until they gain, or regain, reason, and hence the capacity for freely chosen good or evil. So, precisely because the system presupposes the existence of reason, under the terms of its own logic it disqualifies from attention those exemplifications of unreason we term mentally disordered offenders.

Expressed thus, questions about how mentally disordered offenders should be processed raise for consideration the broader question of the legitimacy of an individualised, reason-based structure of justice production and administration. Such a debate presents as a plausible alternative what is, to a society seared by the historical logic of fascism,[5] doubtless an uncomfortable acknowledgement that the system is concerned less with taxonomic questions than with maintaining social order.

To some criminologists, the problem with the rational approach to crime management lies in the metaphysical character of the belief that reason is an acceptable causal explanation of 'normal' crime. To them, as our understanding of the causes of crime increases, our belief in metaphysical explanations will diminish, and we believe misapplied 'reason' is a cause of crime only where there is a vacuum in the biological, human and social sciences. It follows that as scientific understandings increase, the misleading binary divide between responsibility and non-responsibility will shift, and metaphysics yield to more verifiable 'scientific' explanations.

Again, we see that like most theoretical positions, this one has tactical consequences. It leads radical commentators to a belief that punishment should be abolished (Menninger 1968) or transformed into an expression of sorrow and grief (Christie 1981); and conservative ones to a very different conclusion:

> If society should not punish acts that science has shown to have been caused by antecedent conditions, then every advance in knowledge about why people behave as they do may shrink the scope of criminal law. If, for example, it is shown that sex offenders suffer from abnormal hormones combined with certain atypical relations with their parents, then, by the existing standards of responsibility, why should their attorneys not demand acquittal on grounds of bad hormones combined with a particular family history?
>
> (Wilson and Herrnstein 1985: 504–505)

It is plausible to argue that the preferred solution to this conundrum is already evident in the shift of emphasis from courtroom into consulting room and (so-called) community, since in both these loci, ascertaining *mens rea* is of less significance than it is in court. This is not, however, to suggest that we are witnessing the imposition of totalitarian control over the mentally disordered at a time of wholesale closure of those temples of social control, the Victorian mental hospitals. None the less we may assume both that 'the community' will exercise a form of control more diffuse than anything imposed directly by the state (Grant, this volume), and that a key consequence of the increased legitimation of scientific 'understandings' of crime will be the continued expansion of the explanatory and the therapeutic to the point at which we see the marginalisation of the judicial (Moulin 1975). More speculatively, rather as it constituted the thin end of a wedge in the spread of many probation systems (Harris 1995: 55–58), the relative detachment of many juvenile (or youth) court systems from ratiocinatory

approaches to responsibility, and their transformation in many national jurisdictions into sites where expert opinion has near hegemonic status (Harris and
Timms 1993) may – in the longer term – prove a prototype for developments in
the adult system.

One should by no means apologise for the imposition of control over those
whose capacity to damage others is considerable and whose powers of self-
inhibition are limited. It is, however, important to understand that the control
to which such offenders are subject is by no means removed by a decarceration
policy, even where that policy is characterised by neglect and under-funding.
Abandoning minor disordered offenders to a largely self-regulating moral
'community' which, within the limits of law, determines for itself its threshold of
toleration and takes steps to manage situations in which that threshold is exceeded
by the involvement of formal systems, is by no means a strategy devoid of
control. The questions we may choose to ask about it will, however, depend on
what we wish it to achieve. So, if we have a preference for civil liberty over public
order, we shall doubtless reach one conclusion; if we have the opposite predilec-
tion, we shall doubtless reach another. As is almost always the case in the applied
social sciences, one set of theories yields several practical possibilities, dislike of
any one of which, while it never justifies refusing to engage with theory, makes
engaging with the politics of application an urgent imperative.

Justice and order

> Everything works in its own period. Don't you think that people were cured
> by medieval doctors, soaking up black melancholy bile with white saltpetre?
> We could no more use their remedies than they could use ours, but they did
> work once.
>
> (Ackroyd 1993: 83)

Two strands of thought here require disentanglement; or, more precisely,
sequencing, since one derives from the other. First is the question 'what justification exists for a reason-based approach to crime control in a situation in which
pure reason cannot exist?' The political justification is self-evidently that
citizenship rights and personal liberty are bulwarks against state oppression. From
William Penn through John Milton, the Enlightenment philosophers and John
Stuart Mill to the present day, this case is well attested, and in no wise weakened
by the spectacle of the exercise of direct state oppression in countries which
lack this tradition; and it is no part of our wish to disturb this bulwark of civil
liberty. On the contrary, the characteristically British system which so elegantly
synthesises the benefits of statute law with the common law tradition by normally
sentencing on a tariff, but doing so individually and constructively where
appropriate, appears wholly sensible.

But predominantly wise policies and practices can have unintended side-
effects, normally at the interstices; and mentally disordered offenders are nothing

if not interstitial. Hence the second and consequential question is 'how can we conceptualise the control of criminals in varying states of unreason, given the reason-based approach to justice to which we aspire?'

One possibility is indeed to operate as though the disordered were ordered. To do so would have the benefit of avoiding false dichotomies between 'reason' and 'unreason' in a situation in which confidence in the predictive capacity of forensic psychiatry is variable. On the other hand, even if we avoid the Gostin problem – that his approach leaves offenders whose disorder mitigates the harshness of sentence exposed to greater penalty – to proceed thus would be crude. This is partly because assuming rationality where reason is apparently lacking would call the entire system into question (a pragmatic argument, but law is not even primarily a matter of science, and popular endorsement is necessary for its authority to be maintained); partly because it would do little more than transfer yet more power to the very psychiatrists whose capability has been called into question; partly because it is incorrect to assume that because a categorisation may be controversial it is wrong in principle; and partly because to transform an entire system in order to encapsulate more coherently a minority 'hard case' population would be for the tail to wag the dog.

This is not the place to debate whether the belief in the potential of science ultimately to explain all human behaviour is correct, although today we are still some way from a situation in which it can do so, and it would be wrong to base a judicial system on a hypothetical and culturally alien future discovery. We should by no means necessarily strive for the ideal option when the least bad one is good enough. As R.H. Tawney once observed, because absolute cleanliness is impossible, it does not follow that we should wallow in a dunghill; and because, doubtless, no human choice is unconstrained or unaffected by circumstance, it does not follow that it lacks volition, or that alternative choices could not have been made. Equally, because there is an awkward grey area between the extremes of sanity and madness, it does not mean that we cannot exercise sensible judgement in most cases, and argue about the best way forward at the borderlines.

It is, however, helpful for practitioners to be aware of and reflect on the character of the system they are charged with implementing. Rather than just complaining when more funding fails to arrive, for example, they might ask *why* it is that successive governments have proved reluctant to provide a humane and well-resourced set of facilities for a needy population seemingly unnecessarily detained in prison.

Part of the reason for this reluctance must be that it would be a rash government which released the most difficult offenders from secure into semi-secure (or even open or sheltered) custody, for fear of a popular reaction the first time something went wrong. This seems in turn associated with two phenomena: first the notion of madness as 'beyond reason' and therefore immune to the rational discourse with which most of us are comfortable (a point made earlier); and, second, a decided lack of confidence both in clinicians' predictive capacity and in the supervisory efficacy of probation and social services staff. Since many less risky and more popular causes are equally short of resources, in the absence of an improbable heightening of pressure by the Council of Europe or the United Nations, demands for improved facilities for mentally disordered offenders will be mainly restricted to pressure and professional interest groups.

The main source of wider pressure seems likely to entail demands for greater intensity of control of all mentally disordered offenders in the wake of the occasional high-profile serious crimes committed by people inappropriately or unavoidably discharged from custody, or who are at large anyway but suddenly come to public notice. Such demands seldom address the fundamental issues, but only the symptom, seemingly as part of some collective psychological search for meaning out of tragedy; a point exemplified in the introduction of handgun restrictions and improved school security following the Dunblane shootings, as though the danger were the inherently unlikely repetition of a specific problem, not the absence of a broader and more strategic approach to serious crime prevention, or of a capacity to identify and manage dangerous people.

In this chapter, no radically new way forward is offered, and the intellectual blandishments of those who seek scientific explanations of all human wrongdoing are resisted not so much on grounds of superior argument (though this should not be taken as implying that such arguments do not exist – simply that this is not the place in which to air them) as on the pragmatic ground that the cures available show every indication of being worse than the disease:

> The disastrous people are the indelicate and conceited busybodies who want to reform criminals and mould children's characters by external pressure . . . the busybody, the quack, the pseudo God Almighty . . . is the irreconcilable enemy, the ubiquitous and iniquitous nuisance, and the most difficult to get rid of because he has imposed his moral pretensions on public opinion, and is accepted as just the sort of philanthropist our prisons and criminals should be left to.
>
> (George Bernard Shaw 1941: 115–116)

As a characteristic part of Herschel Prins's intellectual contribution has been to urge professionals to think hard about what they are doing – its morality as well as its efficacy – and see things differently and in an un-commonsensical way, this may be no bad place to stop. That our capacity to see problems with what we do comes before our capacity to see what we should be doing instead is no reason to eschew ideas which lack consequential actions. To acknowledge limitations in the current state of knowledge but to proceed notwithstanding in the hope that the actions will follow later is a defensible way forward.

It may well be – in one hundred, two hundred years – that much of what we believe or do today will be shown unequivocally to be wrong. But justice systems have not only to be as 'right' as they can be in the current state of knowledge but to reflect a fair and civilised version of contemporary norms and beliefs, so ensuring political and popular acceptability. This is what the law is and has to do, and it cannot base itself on discoveries yet to be made and which may never be made. It is not only, not even especially, with the law itself, however, but with its implementation by professionals doing their best to be sensible, flexible and self-reflective in a difficult and often confused situation that Herschel Prins's work is concerned; and the contribution of the knowledge and wisdom of the most thoughtful professionals to the reform process seems almost certain to be considerable.

In conclusion

> I think it is high time that we had the grace, humility, and good sense to leave the dealing out of moral retribution to the Supreme Being and to confine mundane efforts to concerns more promisingly and justly within our competence.
>
> (Glueck 1963: 136)

This chapter has not sought to offer new solutions, but to excavate some of those which already exist in the hope that doing so will prepare the way for the efforts of others better equipped to map a way forward. And here at least we have run some quarry to ground, though doubtless many foxes have got away.

First, we have taken as our text the sensitivity of Herschel Prins to the subjective, experiential ways of viewing the world which he sees as necessary contributors to our understanding of the diffuse phenomenon of mental disorder. From this, it follows that the discourse of 'objective science' is – certainly today and perhaps it always will be – an insufficient and possibly a fatally flawed framework for grasping or dealing with mentally disordered offenders.

Second, from this we can come to understand better the seeming bewilderment of judges, politicians and others at the predictive fallibility of the psychiatrists who, far from being engaged in a laboratory-based enterprise of single variable manipulation, are thrown into the unpredictable maelstrom of marginal, often socially excluded, life. In this milieu, clinical, environmental, attitudinal, cognitive, perceptual, behavioural, cultural and economic variables mutate so unpredictably with the comforting disciplines of psychology, sociology, politics, biochemistry and anthropology that one scarcely knows which way to turn. How can one 'choose' just one of these disciplines to comprehend such social anarchy? Yet how can one play 'lucky dip' with all of them without effectively abandoning all pretence at scientific method, all rules of analysis, all belief in a controllable and consistent universe? Should social and human scientists be striving for 'rules of eclecticism', whereby they can produce verifiable (and refutable) procedures for multi-disciplinary endeavours? Or should they abandon such a Promethean endeavour and settle for the experiential, the subjective, the creative and the phenomenological as not only a practical but a theoretically defensible approach?

More to the point, how can one predict the way in which a single individual, subject to almost infinite influences from numerous sources and already probably a marginal, vulnerable and potentially erratic person, will respond to 'life', 'freedom' or 'community control'? One may as well rampage in the chemistry laboratory, randomly emptying phials into a single container, shaking it with abandon and then claiming, without any idea what the constituents are, to know how the resultant compound will react to being set on fire. One can advise on probabilities, but the fact that the bookmaker and his *haut bourgeois* cousin the insurance underwriter will, if they know their business and wait long enough, always win in the end is scarcely good enough for an anxious public. This is hardly surprising, when the concern is not immediately with statistical probability but with a difficult individual whose behaviour – for all the sophistication of contemporary risk assessment tools that increasingly dominate the working ethos of the human service professions – is ultimately unpredictable.

Third, from this we identify two parallel discourses of medico-penal control philosophy, their differences too seldom articulated. The first emphasises the primacy of individual justice. Rooted in the social contract of the Enlightenment philosophers, it draws on rights and duties as the basis of a social organism, with rational men and women eschewing prohibited pleasures for the common good, and in return claiming protection against those who would harm them. When the Constituent Assembly introduced a principle of strict legality into the French Penal Codes of 1791 and 1810, in the belief that the criminal code could never be too precise, creating what Radzinowicz has called 'the iron equation of crime and punishment affirmed by the classical codes' (in Ancel 1971: vii), it was instituting, in the name of justice and equality, an assumptive framework which, in that its bedrock was the assumption of rationality, added greatly to the marginalisation of the insane.

The second discourse, on the other hand, subordinates considerations of individual justice to the common good, acknowledging that, within obvious sensible boundaries, the key to the management of the mentally disordered has only incidentally to do with questions of reason or unreason, and everything to do with the maintenance of public order and security against actually or potentially disordered, and so disruptive, elements. Here, 'reason' is (pejoratively) meta-physical; the main concern is to ensure that disruptive people are controlled, their rights and liberty being subjected to a utilitarian calculus, and necessarily subordinated to the common good.

Fourth, we dismiss the idea that we should seek to secure a conceptualisation of the criminal process so inclusive as to encompass every hard case we encounter. To do so would either produce statements of such generality and abstraction as to be pointless, or would venture into a futuristic world in which all human behaviour will one day be explicable, with reason and choice exposed as outdated theological metaphors. But sometimes a 'good enough' solution is the best to which we can reasonably aspire: we should not, after all, make the perfect the enemy of the good, and it is in particular a misunderstanding of the social function of law to believe that it can depart too far from the very social forces, beliefs and power structures of which it is itself a product.

Fifth, the study of those at the margins can tell us much about those at the mainstream, just as in literature recent contributions from the margins – rediscovered women writers, black writers, working-class writers and writers of new literatures in English in particular – have offered a critique of the mainstream culture the more powerful because it emerges from the interstices. To look in from the margins tells us not so much anything that is new about the marginal activity itself (which may well be of limited interest other than to those committed to the advancement of this or that good cause), but much that is new about the assumptions which underpin our understanding of the mainstream. And, as we said at the beginning, this chapter, which like this book, is about marginal people, is itself written from the margins, by an outsider who has discovered, in the course of researching it, things he has found both interesting and surprising, and which have led him to view his own specialisms in a slightly different way.

Sixth, we have had harsh words for the word 'community'. It is a comforting word, redolent of interdependence and mutuality, though in this context it seems to mean merely 'not locked up'. But to imply that those social inadequates we term mentally disordered offenders, left to fend for themselves in an unlovely array of common lodging houses, soup kitchens and hostels, are somehow in the bosom of a caring community is not very sensible. Nor, given that their mental disorder is such as to exonerate them from responsibility for criminality, does it seem logical to believe them none the less sufficiently 'together' to fend for themselves in an inhospitable and dangerous world with which few of us, for all our supposed intelligence or resourcefulness, would be able to cope.

Seventh, this neglect is by no means the polar opposite of control, albeit that the control in question is diffuse and unpredictable, involving, for each offender, a unique combination of self- and other-control. 'Community care' entails individual deviance being held at a level of tolerance acceptable to those with whom the offender interacts, with deviance beyond that level causing help to be sought from formal control systems. This, of course, enables the costly expertise of the professionals to be targeted at cases which cause visible social problems, and not to be wasted on cases which can be contained in open conditions at little or no financial cost.

But once we accept that there is no pure reason, then nor can there be pure madness; only shades of grey. And just as people we perceive 'fundamentally good' prove capable of bad acts, and people we perceive 'fundamentally bad' prove capable of good ones (thereby destroying at a stroke the very bases of their attributed characters), and once we are startled by some uncharacteristic 'act of madness' committed by the most normal of people, we are some way down the path to challenging the categories themselves, and accepting our role, as well as that of the mentally disordered, as parts of a complex and perhaps ultimately impenetrable humanity.

This is a theoretical point, and human action cannot be driven by theory alone. Accordingly, the necessity of classification is beyond question, and it need not matter that history will one day tell us that we have got the classifications wrong.

That fine judgements honestly made are necessary at the borderlines can similarly be taken as read; so can the fact that a relativistic concept such as 'diminished responsibility' is in application translated into a binary divide which makes little sense in psychiatric, but perfect sense in legal theory. Let us not make the perfect the enemy of the good, and let us not give undue weight to one discourse over competing ones.

In looking again at mentally disordered offenders, it can, as Herschel Prins might remind us, be helpful to ponder – with some humility – whether we academic or professional observers are confident that we are ourselves so mentally ordered as to be incapable of moments of madness; and that our most sane acts are never driven by motives other than those we plausibly represent as their cause. To Herschel Prins the world is a messy and unpredictable place, but everyone, professionals and scholars as well as the offenders, deviants or patients who provide those professionals and scholars with a better living than they themselves could ever dream of, has to do his or her best to get by decently, and to try to do more good than harm along the way. This seems an honourable aim, and one which Herschel Prins, though he would never admit or even think it, has himself indubitably met.

Notes

1 The author is grateful to Anita Gibbs and Roger Statham for their helpful comments on an earlier draft of this chapter.
2 For discussions of more general developments here, see Higgins (1994); Walker (1985: Chapter 21); Hoggett (1990); Walker (1991); Peay (1994).
3 The subtitle of this book, taken from the transcript of an interview with a respondent asked to define 'secure accommodation' was *Between Hospital and Prison or Thereabouts*.
4 Of course, when the mentally disordered offenders are also women they can constitute a case study in double marginality, with the boundary between sanity and insanity set rather differently (see, for example, Allen 1987; Peay 1994: 1139–1140).
5 Fascism being a political philosophy by no means confined to Germany but, at least until the exposure of the Holocaust in the mid-1940s, culturally consonant with much Western intellectual thought (Carey 1992).

References

Ackroyd, P. (1993) *The House of Doctor Dee*. London: Hamish Hamilton.
Allen, H. (1987) *Justice Unbalanced: Gender, Psychiatry and Judicial Decisions*. Milton Keynes: Open University Press.
Ancel, M. (1971) *Suspended Sentence*. London: Heinemann Educational Books.
Blackburn, R. (1993) *The Psychology of Criminal Conduct: Theory, Research and Practice*. Chichester: John Wiley.
Carey, J. (1992) *The Intellectuals and the Masses: Pride and Prejudice among the Literary Intelligentsia, 1880–1939*. London: Faber & Faber.
Christie, N. (1981) *Limits to Pain*. Oxford: Martin Robertson.
Craft, M. (1984) 'Predicting dangerousness and future convictions among the mentally

abnormal'. In M. Craft and A. Craft (eds) *Mentally Abnormal Offenders*. London: Baillière Tindall.

Craft, M. and Craft, A. (eds) (1984) *Mentally Abnormal Offenders*. London: Baillière Tindall.

Feldman, P. (1977) *Criminal Behaviour: A Psychological Analysis*. London: John Wiley.

—— (1993) *The Psychology of Crime*. Cambridge: Cambridge University Press.

Floud, J. and Young, W. (1981) *Dangerousness and Criminal Justice*. London: Heinemann.

Gerber, P. (1984) 'Psychiatry in the dock: a lawyer's afterthoughts'. In M. Craft and A. Craft (eds) *Mentally Abnormal Offenders*. London: Baillière Tindall.

Glueck, S. (1963) *Law and Psychiatry: Cold War or Entente Cordiale?* London: Tavistock Publications.

Gostin, L. (1984) 'Towards the development of principles for sentencing and detaining mentally abnormal offenders'. In M. Craft and A. Craft (eds) *Mentally Abnormal Offenders*. London: Baillière Tindall.

Grounds, A. (1991) 'The transfer of sentenced prisoners to hospital – 1960–1983'. *British Journal of Criminology*, 31 (1), 54–71.

Gunn, J. (1991) 'The trials of psychiatry: insanity in the twentieth century'. In K. Herbst and J. Gunn (eds) *The Mentally Disordered Offender*. Oxford: Butterworth-Heinemann in association with the Mental Health Foundation.

Harris, R. (1995) 'Probation round the world: origins and development'. In K. Hamai, R. Villé, R. Harris, M. Hough and U. Zvekic (eds) *Probation Round the World: A Comparative Study*. London: Routledge.

Harris, R. and Timms, N. (1993) *Secure Accommodation in Child Care: Between Hospital and Prison or Thereabouts*. London: Routledge.

Heidensohn, F. (1994) 'Gender and crime'. In M. Maguire, R. Morgan and R. Reiner (eds) *The Oxford Handbook of Criminology*. Oxford: Clarendon Press.

Higgins, J. (1984) 'The mentally abnormal offender and his society'. In M. Craft and A. Craft (eds) *Mentally Abnormal Offenders*. London: Baillière Tindall.

—— (1994) 'The mentally disordered offender and his society'. In M. Craft and A. Craft (eds) *Mentally Disordered Offenders*. London: Baillière Tindall.

Hoggett, B. (1990) *Mental Health Law*. 3rd edition. London: Sweet and Maxwell.

Hollin, C. (1989) *Psychology and Crime: An Introduction to Criminological Psychology*. London: Routledge.

Home Office and Department of Health and Social Security (1975) *Report of the Committee on Mentally Abnormal Offenders*. (The Butler Report). Cmnd. 6244. London: HMSO.

Mace, A. (1991) 'A probation service perspective'. In K. Herbst and J. Gunn (eds) *The Mentally Disordered Offender*. Oxford: Butterworth-Heinemann in association with the Mental Health Foundation.

Menninger, K. (1968) *The Crime of Punishment*. New York: The Viking Press.

Moir, A. and Jessel, D. (1995) *A Mind to Crime: The Controversial Link between the Mind and Criminal Behaviour*. London: Michael Joseph.

Moulin, P. (1975) 'Extenuating circumstances'. In M. Foucault (ed.) *I, Pierre Rivière, Having Slaughtered my Mother, my Sister, and my Brother . . . : A Case of Parricide in the 19th Century*. (trans. F. Jellinek). Lincoln: University of Nebraska Press.

Mustill, M. (1991) 'Some concluding reflections'. In K. Herbst and J. Gunn (eds) *The Mentally Disordered Offender*. Oxford: Butterworth-Heinemann in association with the Mental Health Foundation.

Norrie, A. (1986) 'Practical reasoning and criminal responsibility: a jurisprudential approach'. In D.B. Cornish and R.V. Clarke (eds) *The Reasoning Criminal: Rational Choice Perspectives on Offending*. New York: Springer-Verlag.

Peay, J. (1994) 'Mentally disordered offenders'. In M. Maguire, R. Morgan and R. Reiner (eds) *The Oxford Handbook of Criminology*. Oxford: Clarendon Press.

Pinder, M. and Laming, H. (1991) 'Time to re-think'. In K. Herbst and J. Gunn (eds) *The Mentally Disordered Offender*. Oxford: Butterworth-Heinemann in association with the Mental Health Foundation.

Prins, H. (1986) *Dangerous Behaviour, the Law and Mental Disorder*. London: Tavistock Publications.

—— (1995) *Offenders, Deviants or Patients?* 2nd edition. London: Routledge.

Radzinowicz, L. and Turner, J. (eds) (1944) *Mental Abnormality and Crime: Introductory Essays*. London: Macmillan.

Shaw, G.B. (1941) *The Crime of Punishment*. New York: Philosophical Library.

Staite, C., Martin, N., Bingham, M. and Daly, R. (1994) *Diversion from Custody for Mentally Disordered Offenders*. Harlow: Longman Information and Reference.

United Nations (1988) *Body of Principles for the Protection of All Persons Under Any Form of Detention or Imprisonment*. Resolution 43/173. New York: United Nations.

Walker, N. (1985) *Sentencing: Theory, Law and Practice*. London: Butterworth.

—— (1991) 'Fourteen years on'. In K. Herbst and J. Gunn (eds) *The Mentally Disordered Offender*. Oxford: Butterworth-Heinemann in association with the Mental Health Foundation.

Wilson, J.Q. and Herrnstein, R. (1985) *Crime and Human Nature: The Definitive Study of the Causes of Crime*. New York: Simon & Schuster.

Chapter 2

Public Inquiries in mental health

(with particular reference to the Blackwood case at Broadmoor and the patient-complaints of Ashworth Hospital)

Louis Blom-Cooper

Preamble

The time is ripe for informed public debate about the circumstances in which inquiries should or should not be instituted into problems which arise with the management of mentally disordered offenders in institutional settings. In particular, attention should be paid to the most appropriate means of striking the difficult balances between such conflicting pulls as respecting personal privacy while at the same time ensuring that the cleansing effect of public scrutiny is applied to a situation which has gone badly wrong. This chapter contributes to that debate, arguing for an approach which is not, I know, favoured by Herschel Prins. If, in the course of putting my case, anything I have written strikes an overly critical or discordant note, it must nevertheless not be read as detracting from the respect and scholarly regard in which I hold Herschel Prins.

Disagreement between professional colleagues is the life blood of sensible social discourse. For nearly half a century, Herschel Prins has contributed hugely as an academic, field worker, member of a Mental Health Review Tribunal and member of the Mental Health Act Commission, and writer on the manifold issues relating to the plight of the mentally disordered. It is a privilege to contribute to a volume of essays to celebrate his seventieth birthday.

Public and private inquiries

Herschel Prins spoke at a conference which took place at Brunel University in July 1997 of the work he had undertaken in chairing a Committee of Inquiry into the death of Orville Blackwood in Broadmoor Special Hospital: 'We were not examining individual complaints or blame; instead we were examining patterns of practice within Broadmoor' (Prins 1998: 76). This was consistent with the Report of the Committee of Inquiry in question, which had said: 'Our criticisms, where we have them, are aimed more at practice and custom rather than at individuals' (Committee of Inquiry into the Death in Broadmoor Hospital of Orville Blackwood and a Review of the Deaths of Two Other Afro-Caribbean Patients 1993 [hereinafter the Blackwood Inquiry Report]: 3). The Report itself stemmed from the decision, taken in September 1991 by the Special Hospitals Service Authority (SHSA), to set up a Committee under Herschel Prins's chairmanship.

Orville Blackwood, a young Afro-Caribbean patient at Broadmoor Hospital, had died on 28 August 1991 in a seclusion room in the special care unit. The cause of death, as given by the forensic pathologist, was 'cardiac failure associated with the administration of phenothiazine drugs'. The Inquiry, in addition to examining the circumstances surrounding Blackwood's death, was also asked to examine whether there were any common factors between his death and that of two other young Afro-Caribbean patients who had previously died in seclusion rooms at Broadmoor, Michael Martin, who had died in 1984, and Joseph Watts who had died in August 1988.

This decision to institute the Blackwood Inquiry followed only months on from a decision taken the previous April by the Secretary of State for Health, at the direct instigation of the SHSA, to set up an inquiry to investigate allegations of improper care and treatment of patients at Ashworth Hospital. This latter Inquiry, which was chaired by the present author,[1] was put on a statutory footing by the Secretary of State following a threatened lack of cooperation by the Prison Officers Association, which at that time had a majority of the nursing staff in the Special Hospitals in membership. In the case of Ashworth, the allegations of improper care or ill-treatment stemmed from a Channel 4 documentary which had been transmitted on 4 March 1991. In the event, the Ashworth Hospital Inquiry decided to investigate four individual cases in depth, rather than canvass a vast volume of complaints lodged with the authorities over a number of years. The Committee of Inquiry's terms of reference also specifically required a review of arrangements for handling complaints by or on behalf of patients about their care and treatment at Ashworth.

The four cases were:

- Sean Walton, who had died suddenly and unexpectedly in seclusion on 1 March 1988, resulting from the cardiotoxic effect of the drug Pimozide. Combined with physical and emotional arousal, this triggered off cardiac arrhythmia, causing instantaneous death.
- Geoffrey Steele, who had been assaulted by three male nurses in an incident in the ward kitchen on 14 May 1990, as a result of which he had received multiple bruising.
- Gillian Darnell, whose complaint of a sexual assault by a male nurse in March 1985, while it had been found to be believable, was considered not fully proved.
- Gary Harrington, who had committed suicide on 1 May 1990 by hanging himself in his room, seemingly a predictable and preventable happening.

(Report of the Committee of Inquiry into Complaints about Ashworth Hospital 1992 [Volume II])

The four cases constituted a focus for a consideration of the Hospital's care and treatment (or lack of it) of patients. Similarly, Chapter 7 of Herschel Prins's Blackwood Report focused on the day of Orville Blackwood's death, describing (without assigning or apportioning blame for the incident) how the nurses had restrained Blackwood and asked the doctor (who, though anonymous in the Report, was readily identifiable) what to do: 'He decided to administer Sparine 150mg intramuscularly to act as an immediate sedative. He also ordered the administration of Modecate 150mg intramuscularly for the long-term control of the patient's psychosis' (Blackwood Inquiry Report 1993: 30).

The Report did, however, address the question of lack of care and treatment. While rejecting a charge of ill-treatment of patients within the meaning of section 127 of the Mental Health Act 1983, the Committee did conclude, without singling out any one member of the medical or nursing staff, that:

> there were occasions when the care given to Orville Blackwood could and should have been of a higher standard . . . Orville Blackwood's primary nurse did not know the patient at all. This caused us a great deal of concern. None of the staff in the special care unit appear (*sic*) to have really got to know Orville Blackwood . . . After careful consideration of the evidence we could find nothing to substantiate claims that Orville Blackwood was either victimised or physically abused during his stay at Broadmoor Hospital.
>
> (Blackwood Inquiry Report 1993: 26–27)

The Committee turned its main attention to a number of themes relating to hospital management and regimes. It asserted that there was no overt racism within Broadmoor Hospital, but that indirect and unconscious racism remained a minor problem. It discussed the medication administered, and made some helpful recommendations. It decided that the seclusion of Blackwood had been wrong, though understandable; the decision 'was an over-reaction to a patient unwilling to conform to a rigid, structured regime. It was the wrong decision, an automatic conflict-response' (ibid.: 33). The Committee was critical of the size of the Special Care Unit, but rejected any link between the deaths of Blackwood, Martin and Watts. It made some helpful comments about the use of control and restraint techniques and had important things to say about organisational issues, such as medical leadership and lines of medical responsibility.

Does this analysis of a public inquiry differ from that indicated by the Ashworth Hospital Inquiry? Apart from the description of the four cases which were dealt with extensively in Volume II of the Report in a manner designed to provide the specialist reader with the *minutiae* of the case histories, the same thematic issues were covered. Part F of the Report dealt with, *inter alia*, control and restraint, seclusion, medication, deaths in Special Hospitals, patient-family involvement, documentation and hospital records. While none of the four patients came from any ethnic minority, the Committee nevertheless concluded that 'the culture at Ashworth nurtures covert and fosters overt racism', a topic to which the Committee had devoted one of its seminars, and which, as we have seen, also surfaced as a theme in Herschel Prins's Inquiry, where, although a different conclusion was reached, nevertheless:

> compared with the problem of overt racist attitudes and literature of Ashworth Hospital . . . the problems are minor . . . there is a problem, and the problem is with staff attitudes. We therefore conclude that there is racism in Broadmoor Hospital. It is not on the whole deliberate or necessarily conscious, there was some evidence of direct racism in some areas.
>
> (Blackwood Inquiry Report 1993: 55)

Thus, both inquiries were set up and designed to allay public disquiet about the propriety of the kind of care and treatment accorded to patients detained contemporaneously in two of the three Special Hospitals managed and operated by the Special Hospital Services Authority, both before and after the SHSA's inception in October 1989. Without dilating unnecessarily on the issue, one can and may conclude that both Committees were examining patterns of practice within the two hospitals in order to set the scene, differing only in their emphasis on individual complaints or blameworthiness on the part of the actors in the hospital setting.

For these reasons, the particular events under scrutiny at Broadmoor and Ashworth raise many of the same questions about the conduct of a public inquiry in the mental health field. In truth and in essence, public disquiet about the running of the Special Hospitals was precisely the same: events happened – detained patients under the Mental Health Act 1983 had died or been maltreated in closed institutions under the same management. A number of issues immediately pose themselves. For example, should such inquiries be held in private or in public? What is the most effective way of ensuring that what in fact happened (as well as why and how) is accurately established by the inquiry process? Can the process be conducted without the injection of bias and prejudice? What role (if any) do the families of the victims of homicides (and lesser criminal offences) and the communities in which disturbing events occur have in the process? Does it suffice that the inquiry report is published? How does one balance the wish to protect those under scrutiny from the ordeal of public accountability and answerability, with the public wish to be reassured that what happened will not recur?

The questions can be sensibly answered only if the framework for the public inquiry is first understood. Some basic facts need to be stated. The Ashworth Committee sat between September 1991 and January 1992 on 37 days and heard evidence from 83 different witnesses. In March 1992 it held seminars on 14 selected topics over 10 days. Between January and March 1992, two experts on nursing carried out an audit at Ashworth to report on the hospital regime then operative, compared with the time of the incidents involving the four cases. The Committee reported to the Secretary of State for Health in July 1992, submitting a two volume report. Volume I contained 261 pages, with a selected bibliography, appendices of 128 pages and an index of 37 pages; Volume II contained 101 pages. The whole exercise, from the date of appointment, took just under 15 months.

Herschel Prins's Committee was set up in September 1991, and the Inquiry team met for the first time shortly thereafter. It met on 19 occasions to take oral evidence in private from 50 witnesses, and on 7 further occasions to consider the issues and formulate its report, completion of which was delayed partially by the second inquest into Orville Blackwood's death, held from 29 March to 2 April 1993 and confirming the verdict of accidental death (though the Committee did not wait to see a full transcript of the coroner's proceedings). The Report is 81 pages long, with two annexes of 6 pages. It contains no index, but includes a summary and a list of recommendations. It reported in August 1993, so taking nearly two years from start to finish, though as an instance of inordinate delay, the report of the *Luke Warm Luke* Mental Health inquiry, presented to Lambeth, Southwark and Lewisham Health Authority on 13 November 1998, takes the biscuit. This took just over three years from the setting up of the three-member inquiry under the chairmanship of Baroness Scotland of Asthal QC, to the date of publication (also known as 'The Scotland Report').

Neither the Blackwood Report, nor that into the complaints at Ashworth Hospital discloses the cost to the public purse, but it must be assumed that the Ashworth Inquiry was infinitely more costly, not least in the light of the payment to legal representatives of fees out of public funds. There's the rub. The Broadmoor Inquiry met in private and, in the words of the Report itself, informally. Oral witnesses were questioned in what was tantamount to a private meeting, when, though they were invited to bring a friend or legal adviser, the Committee 'took evidence from the witnesses only'. The Ashworth Committee of Inquiry, on the other hand, after having studied a vast amount of documentary material which disclosed a worrying state of affairs, decided to conduct oral hearings in public. Apart from two counsel to the Inquiry, some 16 counsel appeared for a number of witnesses (one counsel representing all the patient-complainants). At all stages, the parties' legal representatives were permitted to ask questions under the strict control of the Chairman. The permitted style was more that of questioning than of cross-examination.

In their Report, referring pointedly to other inquiries where lawyers were actively engaged, Herschel Prins and his colleagues claimed that:

> the way in which we conducted our Inquiry led to a greater free exchange of information and opinion, unrestricted by the adversarial atmosphere that pertains at public, judicial or quasi-judicial inquiries. We were able to proceed in this manner because we were not investigating specific complaints or allegations. We were examining policy and procedures within Broadmoor Special Hospital.
>
> (Blackwood Inquiry Report 1993: 3)

But the mere fact that potential criticism is directed at policies and practices rather than at individuals provides no answer to the question of legal representation; nor does it necessarily determine the atmosphere of the proceedings. Criticism is presumably no less painful to the policy-maker and practitioner because it is primarily aimed at policy and practice, and it is surely a delusion to believe that the one can be dissociated from the other. Fairness – which, together with thoroughness, form the two *desiderata* of any public inquiry – will always encompass the purveyors of policy and practice. There may be a sharing of collective responsibility which will no doubt soften the individual's pain of critical examination, but each one will feel, none the less, the need to be protected against unjust criticism. Whether the strength of that feeling is sufficient to justify legal representation may be questionable, but the need for protection cannot be gainsaid. And the legalism of public inquiries is anyway highly debatable: a debate on this very point raged around the Scott Inquiry into Arms for Iraq – which was also more about Government policies, ministerial actions and practices of the civil service than about the conduct of individuals, and is still the subject of heated contention (I return to the Scott Inquiry later).

The assertion that the absence of legal representatives and the adversarial system leads to 'a free exchange of information and opinion' is unsubstantiated by any experience of the two systems. The injection of legalism into any forum of investigation can often be elucidating as well as confounding. (Lawyers are – or ought to be – adept at sifting out the relevant from the irrelevant or peripheral issues. Appropriately controlled by the inquiring body, the legal input can facilitate both the process and the outcome of a report.) A witness who can give evidence about events and people without direct questioning from those affected adversely by his or her testimony is capable of distortion or misrepresentation, not to say lying. If conducted in private, the problem raised by this lack of protection against false information is all the greater. While a transcript of the witnesses' statement or oral testimony – it is not clear whether the Broadmoor Inquiry provided everyone with a record of what was said – will go some way towards remedying any manifest unfairness in the process, there is really no escape from the requirement that an individual who is or is liable to be criticised should have a full opportunity to meet that criticism, if necessary through the medium of the advocate. If that opportunity cannot be provided during the inquiry process, there must be an opportunity to see the relevant part(s) of the penultimate version of the report, an opportunity offered, for example, by Sir Richard Scott in the Arms for Iraq Inquiry.

There is, moreover, nothing so adversarial as a probing inquisition; the adversaries are the inquisitors and those whose conduct is being scrutinised. Did Herschel Prins and his colleagues discover (or uncover) a more effective way of arriving at what happened to Orville Blackwood and his two fellow Afro-Caribbeans at Broadmoor than did the authors of the Ashworth Hospital Inquiry into the cases of Walton, Steele, Darnell and Harrington? I do not pause to answer a problematical question. Suffice it to say, the answer does not strike one as obvious, though one thing needs to be said: the Ashworth Hospital Inquiry put in place, as an adjunct to its adversarial process, seminars on 14 topics relating to policy and practices at the Special Hospital – surely nowadays a well-tried method of exchanging information and opinion. The style and pattern of public inquiries are inevitably diffuse and unsettled. Each has to be tailored according to the subject-matter and its terms of reference.

Herschel Prins does, however, have a point, not answered readily by those who favour the more formal process of inquiries. It is the cost. Undoubtedly the Broadmoor Inquiry, without the benefit (or should it be hindrance?) of legal representatives was far less costly to conduct than was Ashworth. There is clearly a need to curtail the cost of lawyers, if not to exclude them from the inquiry process. Sir Richard Scott effectively excluded legal representation at, and during, the hearings in the Arms to Iraq Inquiry, although he conducted the inquisitorial process in a formal manner, and lawyers were able to assist their clients in answering lengthy questionnaires administered by the Inquiry. He used the services of leading counsel in the examination of witnesses, and sat mostly in public. He also provided transcripts and administered comprehensive questionnaires on those due to give evidence. His unusual procedure was not universally applauded. He was excoriated by Lord Howe of Aberavon both in oral exchange during the Inquiry and in learned articles in academic journals and elsewhere (Howe 1994; 1996).

The solution to the problem of legal representation appropriate to inquiries in the mental health field may be found in the BSE Inquiry currently (September 1998) being conducted by Lord Justice Phillips. There the inquiry has been divided into two distinct parts. The first is pure fact-finding. Witnesses are called without the involvement of lawyers. Only as and when the tribunal has found the facts and analysed the evidence does it move to the second stage of examining culpability for what happened. At that stage those liable to be criticised are asked to respond to particular criticism, and permitted to do so through legal representatives. We shall await with interest both the outcome of the Inquiry and the comments of participants in the process.

Public or private?

Herschel Prins is a committed adherent of holding hearings – in whatever style – in private. He asserts that the decision to remain behind closed doors does not 'detract from either veracity or fairness'. His own experience, he claims, has not demonstrated detriment to anyone. These are bold and untested assertions. All one can say is that what an individual may say out of hearing of any adversary who is unable to question the testimony must be inherently unsafe. Why else would the legal system be so insistent on a public process? Those who wish to have their disputes resolved out of public sight have to invoke the system of arbitration. In the institutional setting, conflicts between members of staff are notoriously common; they may find a ready outlet for personal hostility in the inquiry forum. My own experience contradicts Herschel's viewpoint. Of the two child abuse inquiries with which I was involved as Chairman – Jasmine Beckford (Commission of Inquiry into the Circumstances Surrounding the Death of Jasmine Beckford 1985) and Kimberley Carlile (Commission of Inquiry into the Circumstances Surrounding the Death of Kimberley Carlile 1987) – the former was in public, while the latter I was persuaded to conduct in private. Without elaborating, I found the former process incomparably more manageable, with no loss of evidential material. Moreover, while the media reported the public hearing accurately enough, the private inquiry was reported inaccurately as a result of leaks by participants – a highly unsatisfactory situation.

Beyond that, however, if the setting up of an inquiry is prompted by public disquiet, it follows that that disquiet will be best allayed by a full display of the events that caused it. The presumption must, therefore, be in favour of public hearings.

Herschel Prins identifies as the key issue the achievement of fairness to all parties, not least the personnel under scrutiny, and cites the moving account, given at a recent conference, by the Responsible Medical Officer, Dr Ray Goddard, in the Jason Mitchell Inquiry (Blom-Cooper et al. 1996). The inquiry was 'clearly a traumatic experience, for even if no blame attaches, the professional is likely to feel, perhaps quite irrationally, that he or she is likely to blame' (Prins 1998: 80). The SHSA, in its response to the Report, concluded that:

> some of the report's findings may be painful for the individuals involved and for the organisation as a whole, but unexpected deaths such as these made it necessary to examine the hospital's work . . . Publication of this report is part of the openness we want to promote throughout the Special Hospitals Service.

It was in somewhat similar words that the Director of Security for the SHSA told the Ashworth Hospital Committee of Inquiry 'It is always a painful sort of process to have your own organisation looked at.' Herschel Prins adds that pain is less bearable if the hearings are in public. But that can only be so because of the wider audience, surely a slight exacerbation only of the pain resulting from a self-perceived failure in professional work.

Any scrutiny of the conduct of professional or other services is at best uncomfortable and at worst painful, but the worst aspect of Dr Goddard's experience in the Jason Mitchell Inquiry was the grossly inaccurate report and unjust accusation made by a national newspaper on the day in July 1995 that Jason Mitchell was sentenced at Ipswich Crown Court for the manslaughter of his father and the Wilsons. Everything said and done thereafter in the ensuing inquiry served only to soften that initial widely disseminated impact. If the inquiry had been held in private, correction would have had to wait nine months, to the day of the publication of the Report in March 1996. Dr Goddard demonstrably suffered an unpleasant experience in December 1994 following his patient's horrendous deed. Palpably, as time wore on, he was able to accommodate the rigours of the inquiry process with increasing assuredness and even, by the end of the hearings, with self-composure. In any event, those who provide professional services in the public sector must expect to be answerable in the most public way. They have to stand up and be counted, as Sir Richard Scott said in justifying his public hearings involving potential criticism of civil servants.

All those whose lives are touched, either directly or even peripherally, by the inquiry process deserve to have their privacy and occupations respected. But above all, the victims are not just those who come under public scrutiny. The events which are the subject of inquiry leave their own trail of victims – the mentally disordered offender who kills, his or her family and friends, the families of the victims of the homicide, as well as the local community which will contain many people likely to be disturbed psychologically by the tragedy in their midst. A whole closely-knit village may be profoundly affected. They too are not left untouched by what is revealed in the Inquiry.

The families of the victims typically have two overriding concerns – first, they feel a burning need to know precisely what happened and how and why it came about, even if the process of learning may at the time be compounding their ordeal of bereavement and pain; second, they need assurance that what happened to them or their family will not happen to others. Those concerns are best met by the openness of the inquiry process. One has only to read the statement made by Christopher Wilson (on behalf of himself and his two sisters) to the Jason Mitchell Inquiry to appreciate these concerns. And what about the local populace? The Chairman of Suffolk Health Authority, Mrs Joanna Spicer, spoke for the electorate of East Suffolk when she said in a statement that, unless there was some overriding reason for holding an Inquiry in private, there should be a presumption of publicity.

Two things perhaps need to be added. First, the question whether an inquiry should be in public should be determined by the sponsoring authority, not the members of the inquiry team: that is to say, the terms of reference should declare the mode of inquiry (this was done in the Jason Mitchell case). Second, there needs to be a much more sophisticated system of sieving, to determine which homicidal and other serious events call for a given level of investigation. Many, if not most of the inquiries in the mental health field require no more than internal inquiry; a few call for some outside, independent inquiry without the panoply of a full-scale collation of evidence and a detailed report; still fewer – a handful perhaps – require the genuine article of a public inquiry in order to respond appropriately to pronounced public disquiet about an actual or perceived scandal or disaster. It may be that the three deaths at Broadmoor did not arouse such public disquiet as to merit the full treatment of openness. Ashworth certainly did. The Scotland Report (1998) makes two helpful recommendations about public inquiries. It urges Government to re-examine the scope and subject matter of inquiries; and it suggests the publication of a Handbook on Inquiries to guide the participants through the thickets of procedural issues.

The plethora of public inquiries in the field of mental health, however conducted, will each have contributed to a shift in official policy in emphasis on community care to the provision of 'asylum' (in the best sense of the word) for some mentally disordered people who find life in the real world discombobulating, if not entirely disagreeable. Perhaps with some thought of this kind in his mind, Herschel Prins concluded his paper on inquiries into untoward deaths in the mental health system with a quotation from Dr Adrian Grounds of the Cambridge Institute of Criminology with which I heartily concur. Accordingly, I conclude my own contribution in precisely the same way:

> Psychiatric scandals are important levers of long-term reforms. The prevailing criticism of psychiatry in our age is not its excess of social control, but its failures of social control and public protection . . . at the present time it may be the voices of families and victims that are prophetic in showing where we need to move, as they articulate a need for services more sensitive to their concerns, and a need for changes in professional attitudes that may be taken for granted in a generation's time.
>
> (Grounds 1997)

Note

1 The Chairman and the three other members of the Inquiry were all serving members of the Mental Health Act Commission, but were appointed in their personal capacity.

References

Blom-Cooper, L., Grounds, A., Guinan, P., Parker, A. and Taylor, M. (1986) *The Case of Jason Mitchell: Report of the Independent Panel of Inquiry*. London: Duckworth.

Commission of Inquiry into the Circumstances Surrounding the Death of Jasmine Beckford (1985) *A Child in Trust*. Brent: London Borough of Brent.

Commission of Inquiry into the Circumstances Surrounding the Death of Kimberley Carlile (1987) *A Child in Mind: Protection of Children in a Responsible Society*. Greenwich: London Borough of Greenwich.

Committee of Inquiry into Complaints about Ashworth Hospital, August 1992. Cm. 2028-I and II. London: HMSO.

Committee of Inquiry into the Death in Broadmoor Hospital of Orville Blackwood and a Review of the Deaths of Two Other Afro-Caribbean Patients (1993) (Blackwood Inquiry Report). *Big, Black and Dangerous?* London: Special Hospitals Service Authority.

Committee of Inquiry into the Case of Luke Warm Luke (1998). London: Lambeth, Southwark and Lewisham Health Authority

Grounds, A. (1997) 'Commenting on inquiries: who needs them?' *Psychiatric Bulletin*, 21, 134–135.

Howe, Lord of Aberavon (1994) 'Scott's salami tactics'. *The Times*, 1 March.

—— (1996) 'Procedure of the Scott Inquiry'. *Public Law*, 445–460.

Prins, H. (1998) 'Untoward deaths in Special Hospital care: implications of these and other inquiries'. In A. Liebling (ed.) *Deaths of Offenders: The Hidden Side of Justice.* Proceedings of a Conference held at Brunel University, Uxbridge, July 1997. Winchester: Waterside Press, on behalf of the Institute for the Study and Treatment of Delinquency.

Chapter 3

The police and the mentally disordered in the community

Philip Bean

At a time when the number of patients in hospitals is falling and those in the community rising it is no accident that the police have become key figures in the delivery of community mental health services. What was once a relatively unimportant feature of mental health legislation – a provision under Section 136 of the Mental Health Act 1983 whereby a police constable has power to remove a mentally disordered person in a public place to a place of safety – has now assumed greater importance. Often, these patients are what Herschel Prins has called the 'unloved, the unlovely and the unlovable' (Prins 1993: 4), and they pose problems not easy to resolve. Like it or not, some means are required to identify and detain them if only to bring them to the attention of those who would care for them. And some organisation must be responsible for that process.

The main powers of detention and treatment for non-offender patients are in Sections 2, 3 and 4 of the Mental Health Act 1983; these sections allow patients to be seen and assessed in their own homes, or elsewhere in private accommodation. Additional provision is required to deal with those mentally disordered in a public place; hence Section 136 of the Mental Health Act 1986, full details of which appear in at the end of this chapter.[1]

Briefly, however, under this section a constable has the power to remove a mentally disordered person (to be called a patient or suspect from now on) to a place of safety in order that the patient be examined by a medical practitioner and interviewed by an approved social worker (ASW) if:

- it appears that the patient is in immediate need of care and control, *and*
- if the constable thinks it is necessary to do so in the person's interests or for the protection of others.

A person moved to a place of safety may be detained for up to 72 hours.

Section 136 provides a means whereby the patient can be assessed and a decision made as to outcome – which may but need not involve compulsory hospitalisation under Sections 2 or 3. This means it is not an admission order, nor does it provide powers for treatment as under Sections 2 and 3. On the face of it, Section 136 appears a straightforward provision aimed at complementing powers found elsewhere; yet for a number of reasons it remains controversial.

Legal and procedural objections

Though a 'place of safety' is defined in Section 135(6)[2] and the choice of the place of safety rests with the police, there is little by way of case law to provide legal benchmarks. What, for example, is 'a place to which the public has access' (or a 'public place' under the 1959 Act)? Jones (1991) reports that a Divisional Court held that 'places to which the public have access' include premises where there are no barriers or notices restricting access, and places to which members of the public have open access, or access if payment is made, or access at certain times of the day (for example, a football stadium) (Jones 1991: 219). But somewhat controversially, the Mental Health Act Commission notes occasions when the police, called to a disturbed individual in a hospital Accident and Emergency department, have declined to use Section 136 on the ground that this does *not* constitute a 'public place' (Mental Health Act Commission 1993: 45).

And there are numerous uncertainties with immediate operational implications. To how many places of safety can the patient be taken? Can a police officer, for example, use a police station as a place of safety and then bring the patient to a hospital for assessment? Can the hospital be a second place of safety, and would detention in this second place of safety be lawful? Jones says not, claiming that no power exists under this section to transfer the patient from one place of safety to another because the main purpose of invoking this section is to detain the patient there (Jones 1991: 220). If this is correct, it puts the police in some difficulty, encouraged as they are not to use a police station, which can become a staging post whilst negotiating with other agencies, including hospitals. Not surprisingly therefore, the Royal College of Psychiatrists believes 'there is a need to review the circumstances under which it may be acceptable, even desirable, to transfer somebody from one Place of Safety to another in order to complete an assessment' (Royal College of Psychiatrists 1997: 18).

Again, when does the 72 hours assessment begin? At the time of arrival at the place of safety or when the patient was first detained? The Mental Health Act Commission says the former (Mental Health Act Commission 1993: para. 10.7(c)), but others may disagree. And how many assessments can be undertaken? Suppose, for example, that a patient is held in a place of safety and seen by a Responsible Medical Officer (RMO) as required by the Act, who says the patient is not mentally disordered. Are the police entitled to seek the views of a second RMO, and a third and a fourth until an RMO does what they want? Probably not, but it is not clear, and this and other legal matters need to be tidied up. After all, they are not new powers; similar provisions existed both under the Lunacy Act 1890 and the Mental Health Act 1959.

It would help, too, if avoidable confusions were eradicated. The Mental Health Act Commission notes that terms like 'appropriate adult' (AA), and the 'procedures for entering private premises for the purpose of Section 135' (Mental Health Act Commission 1993: 45) need attention. Yet these are not the most glaring: the persistent erroneous belief that Section 136 is an admission order similar to Sections 2, 3, and 4 creates greater difficulties. It is not unusual to find a hospital Code of Practice refer to Section 136 and talk of 'admitting the patient under Section 136' when it should be 'making an assessment whilst the patient is detained for assessment under a Place of Safety Order'. This confusion is of long standing (Rogers and Faulkner 1987). When a patient on a place of safety order is dealt with as if he or she had been admitted, no ASW is called and no powers exist to provide treatment unless and until the patient has been correctly admitted.

Police and police stations

There are also procedural issues requiring attention. The fact that the police are involved in whatever form cannot but help criminalise what was intended initially to be a non-criminal matter. Detention in a police station greatly adds to the criminalising process, and as most patients are offenders, this strengthens the notion that Section 136 is solely for them. Whichever way one looks at it, the link with the criminal justice system is pronounced.

A solution favoured by some is to stop the police from using the police station as a place of safety – a legal possibility but difficult to implement, since in the Act a place of safety can include a hospital, police station or any other place willing to receive that person. For example, a Consultation Document issued prior to the 1983 Act suggested that hospitals were preferable to police stations (Department of Health and Social Security 1976) and doubted whether police stations should ever be so used; the influential Home Office Circular 66/90 agreed, saying, 'It is desirable that, wherever possible, the place of safety in which the person might be detained should be a hospital and not a police station' (Home Office 1990: 1); and the equally influential Reed Report, putting it slightly differently, stated that, 'In line with current policy, mentally disordered offenders should wherever possible receive care and treatment from health or social services rather than in the criminal justice system' (Department of Health/Home Office 1992: para 11.1) In this Reed was echoing the views of most governments going back at least to 1976.

Police stations, though rarely suitable as places of safety, are sometimes necessary. The Mental Health Act Commission, in spite of its reservations about the use of police stations for this purpose (Mental Health Act Commission 1993: 45), did not recommend prohibiting their use, stating that identifying a preferred place of safety was a matter for local agreement. In doing so the Commission showed a greater awareness of the complexities of the task than have others, though occasionally some government departments grudgingly accept that there are circumstances in which detention in a police station may be necessary (for example Department of Health and Social Security 1976: para. 2.24). Of course, the unpleasantness of many police stations contrasts with the more favourable experience patients might expect to have in hospital or assessment units set up in suitable premises, but alternative venues are not always available, and if they are, they may not be suitable for all types of patient, especially those who are violent. Police stations, on the other hand, are normally convenient, they offer high levels of security and can contain patients safely for lengthy periods of time. Paradoxically, they also provide patients with additional rights: under the Police and Criminal Evidence Act 1984 (hereafter PACE), patients detained in a police station under Section 136 have rights relating to powers of arrest, including a right of access to legal advice and an entitlement to have an appropriate adult (AA) present during subsequent interviews. That an AA is rarely called, reflects police practices not legal provision (Bean and Nemitz 1993).

The Commission also recognises that it can be inappropriate for assessments to be carried out in a hospital ward prior to admission, or where there are not adequate facilities: 'Some hospitals find difficulty in handling violent individuals during the assessment before they are sectioned and before anti-psychotic medication can begin under the Mental Health Act' (Mental Health Act Commission 1993: 45). The Commission recommends that an agreed policy should exist to determine cases suitable for detention in a police station and those where the provision of specialised Section 136 assessment units in suitable premises and locations should be encouraged; and that purchasers should be urged to include such provision in contracts (ibid.: 45).

Yet developing specialised assessment units is expensive, and staffing them difficult. Suitable surroundings have to be provided for interviews and assessments (National Association for the Care and Resettlement of Offenders 1993), but in the past some have been of poor quality, with low standards of care, dirty and without necessary safety facilities. The Royal College of Psychiatrists makes detailed suggestions as to what in their view is required, recommending in particular (with staff safety especially in mind) that specialised units should have interviewing rooms with two doors opening outwards and an observation window; the College also gives advice on lighting, decor and location ('where egress to public places is prevented by locked doors or by sufficient staffing to ensure safe containment') (Royal College of Psychiatrists 1997: 10), and says, while recognising there is no simple solution, that these units should where possible be linked or accessible to a psychiatric facility (ibid.: 8) There are no data on the numbers of units operating, nor on their quality, size or staffing levels, but to promote the collection of such information and to coordinate policies, the Royal College recommends the development of Local Safety Committees.

Clearly, it is not easy to disentangle the links between Section 136 and police, crime, and criminality, but since the choice of a place of safety is for the police, and a hospital is under no obligation to accept a patient under a place of safety, the chances of excluding the police station are slim indeed. Nor would it be wise to do so, given the type of patients requiring detention. As with almost everything surrounding Section 136, there is a desperate shortage of data, and none is available on offenders or offences, either before or at the time of arrest. However, a study of the use of AAs (Bean and Nemitz 1993) suggested, albeit on the basis of data not collected systematically, that well over 50 per cent of Section 136 detainees were offenders at the time of arrest and that the offences were other than for public order. Moreover, data from an earlier MIND study (Rogers and

Faulkner 1987) show that patients detained under Section 136 were mainly chronic, with long histories of compulsory hospitalisation and serious offending.

The association with crime would be less powerful if another occupational group could be persuaded to act in the police's stead. The legal possibility exists: Jones, quoting the Butler Committee, argues that the powers under this section extend to persons such as ambulance staff acting under a constable's direction. He reminds us that places of safety can likewise be staffed by people other than the police, and, quoting para. 9.2 of the Butler Report 1975, observes that 'powers of detention given by Section 136(2) are not conferred expressly on the police but are given to any person party to the detention of the disordered person once he has been brought to the Place of Safety' (Jones 1991).

Would any other occupational group take on the task? The answer is surely no. It is difficult to imagine medical or allied professionals operating a 24-hour 7-days-a-week service, detaining people from inner city areas or high rise housing estates in public places, and coping with the associated dangers. The Royal College of Psychiatrists recognises this, but tries for the best of all possible worlds: on the one hand, it says it is inappropriate for the police to manage the mentally ill, yet on the other wants ' the staffing of a place of safety to include the possibility of a maintained police presence to assist in the management of threatened or actual violence' (Royal College of Psychiatrists 1997: 11). Small wonder the Royal College, in anticipating the likely response, adds that 'Local police services will have worries about the time for which these officers would be tied up in by such a policy' (ibid.: 11) – as indeed they would. Keen though the Royal College may be to keep the police at arm's length, it wants them nearby when the trouble starts; it would be surprising if the police fell for this ploy. Incidentally, were Section 136 to be repealed, one could imagine that the police would still detain such patients, probably on a public order offence, in effect operating a surrogate Section 136 service without medical back-up or the safeguards of a place of safety order.

It is perhaps because no other occupational groups want to deal with such patients that criticisms have subsided. Or rather, they have re-emerged in a slightly different form, sometimes more personal and accordingly more difficult to answer. For example, some critics suggest the police are less than capable in the way they identify mental disorder; and a linked but more trenchant criticism is that they lack the sensitivity found amongst other occupational groups. There are other criticisms, more wide-ranging, such as that the culture and philosophy of policing mitigate against dealing with the mentally disordered (Bynoe 1993), and that the police cannot distinguish categories of mental disorder, such as between learning difficulties and mental illness (quoted in Department of Health/Home Office 1992: para. 11.117).

There is little doubt that the police would welcome more training, but not necessarily of the type suggested and not in the form noted above. Certainly they are not trained to recognise mental disorder, but do they need to be? All the evidence suggests they are quite capable of doing so already, especially in its severe forms, without providing the more sophisticated diagnostic labels of some of their professional colleagues (Bean 1980). That is hardly surprising; most people can recognise mental disorder: its stereotypes are learned in childhood and persistently reaffirmed through adult life, and diagnosis at that level does not require a great deal of sophistication. The less severe conditions such as depression or anxiety may prove more difficult and the police may well under-react to these. If so, that would not be surprising: inter-rater reliability of psychiatric diagnoses is not high amongst any professionals, the more so when diagnosing neurotic conditions, so we should not expect it to be high amongst the police.

The Reed Report calls for 'police training which should cover relevant aspects of the Mental Health Act 1983 and the initial identification of suspects who appear to be mentally disordered' (Department of Health/Home Office 1992: para. 11.197). But what does this mean and how would it operate? Is the Committee asking for introductory courses in psychiatry? Presumably yes as it also calls for 'refresher training and joint training with other groups dealing with mentally disordered offenders'. And in the otherwise measured response of the Report of the Royal College of Psychiatrists, it seems it cannot but help getting in on the act: 'Staff in police stations are rarely trained to deal with this situation' it says (Royal College of Psychiatrists 1997: 6).

These criticisms about training, and others about the supposed lack of sensitivity of the police to the mentally disordered can, I suggest, be interpreted as part of the trench warfare dictated by the mind set which separates criminal justice agencies into the 'caring' and the 'authoritarian', the police firmly fixed in the latter. If so, it is time things changed; whether they like it or not, all criminal justice agencies must learn to work together and no single agency can claim a monopoly of sensitivity.

The training most police say they want involves being given information about existing services. That would be neither difficult to introduce nor expensive. They also want specialised units in the police forces able to advise on appropriate pathways to be followed and to help with legal matters. These units need consist of no more than one or two officers, although they could of course be more sophisticated, offering in-service training to custody officers, beat officers and the like, perhaps working in liaison with outside agencies, so developing inter-agency cooperation. Such units would fill in some of the gaps and be of more use than diagnostically oriented introductory training programmes.

One final comment on the so called 'lack of sensitivity' towards the mentally disordered. Data from the MIND research (Rassaby and Rogers 1987; Rogers and Faulkner 1987; Bean et al. 1991) show how badly the police were treated by hospital staff when they took the patients to hospitals on a place of safety order. They were often kept waiting, sometimes for three hours or more, were rarely told the outcome of the medical decision, and sometimes were required to keep the patient in handcuffs whilst the interviews took place – what Rogers calls a clear case of professional dominance (Rogers 1993) and which can also be seen as one of the uglier features of the British class system. These antagonisms were almost ritualised. Whilst they may have little impact on the professionals, they are likely to have a detrimental impact on the patients. Dare one think the unthinkable? Instead of psychiatric training for the police, why not have the police train the psychiatrists? Or, put less provocatively, why not have joint training packages?

Recording Section 136 and police procedures

No national statistics exist on the numbers of Section 136 orders that are made – there were thought to be about 1,600 cases in 1976, and a similar number in 1979 (Bluglass 1984; HMSO 1976) though such figures as there are show a substantial fall in the number of detentions under Section 136 from 920 in 1992–3 to 740 in 1993–4 followed by an increase to 1,220 in 1995–6 (Department of Health 1997). However, almost all orders recorded are made in the Metropolitan District (85 per cent in 1981, for example) (Hoggett 1984). By contrast Nottinghamshire has had 1 recorded Section 136 Order in nearly 40 years, Wales has about 2 or 3 per year, and some police authorities record none at all. The Mental Health Act Commission (1993) correctly suggests that a nationally agreed recording procedure for all Section 136 Orders would assist matters.

This is not to say Section 136 is not used outside the Metropolitan District, rather, that there are simply no local records any more than there is a central recording system. In a study of custody records for the use of appropriate adults (Nemitz 1997) in relation to which the police clearly used their powers under Section 136, records showed numerous patients as having been detained under a place of safety order but not formally recorded as under a Section 136. Where Section 136 was used, or rather where its powers were used, they were without direct reference to the Act. All of which is astonishing given the length of time the legislation has been in operation.

It is often difficult to appreciate how poor have become the recording systems in the mental health field generally (Bean and Nemitz 1993), and clearly those for Section 136 are no different. In our study on the use of the AAs, there was no method of recording Section 136 data, and only the Metropolitan District requires its officers to provide a formal record – hence the bias in existing statistics. The Department of Health reports that one newly created London NHS Trust accounted for 9 per cent (103) of all Section 136 detentions in 1994–5, whereas in the previous year, directly managed Trusts in the equivalent District Health Authority recorded only 15 Orders. Another Trust recorded 46 detentions in 1995–6 under Section 136 and none in 1994–5. The Department of Health said that particular Trust was unable to explain the change (Department of Health 1997: para. 3.6).

Even more disturbing than the lack of statistical information is the lack of understanding about correct practices. In our study in four East Midlands police stations, crossing three police authorities, not only were there no formal records for Section 136, but procedures did not follow those required in the legislation, particularly in that the police surgeon, not the ASW or the psychiatrist, was the first to be called. We regarded this as wrong, not simply in terms of the correct procedures, but in terms of its implications for mentally disordered offenders generally.

What seemed to be happening was that a police officer would bring a patient to the police station on what was a Section 136 order, but without recording it as such. The custody officer would then call a police surgeon to make an assessment of the patient's psychiatric condition, although there was no legal requirement to do so. If the police surgeon identified mental disorder, the custody officer would then call an ASW who would then call a psychiatrist. Of itself, calling the police surgeon was not important, except that the police surgeon rarely identified mental disorder even when the records gave obvious and glaring examples of mental disorder being present. This meant that a large numbers of patients were not being properly assessed. Whether or not as a result of the police surgeon's assessment, the custody officer would act, either by interviewing the suspect as if he had committed an offence or by calling the ASW. Only rarely would the custody officer disagree with the police surgeon.

Similar procedures existed for offenders who were mentally disordered. The police officer would arrest an offender for, say, theft, and later realise the offender was mentally disordered. This would be recorded on the custody records as something like 'Theft/safety order'. Again, the police surgeon would be called, as of course he should be in this case, since the Code of Practice for the Detention Treatment and Questioning of Police Officers issued under Section 66 of PACE requires the Custody Officer to call a police surgeon if a person brought to a police station appears to be suffering from a mental disorder. As with the Section 136 procedures described above, the police surgeon's assessment was almost always accepted. Therefore, the suspect would be charged with the offence, but in the course of this process the police would rarely pass information on the nature of the mental disorder to an ASW, psychiatrist or to the Court. Occasionally, the police surgeon would advise that an ASW should be called, in which case the suspect would be dealt with as if the patient were under a Section 136 – as suggested in Home Office Circular 66/90, which says that where a mentally disordered person has committed an offence, careful consideration should be given to whether prosecution is required in the public interest. While some means of diversion could also operate, this was not common.

In both examples the police surgeon plays a critical and dual role, both as professional adviser to the custody officer determining the course of action taken, and gatekeeper through whom all must pass. In short, custody officers were using the police surgeon as the first line of defence, or as one custody officer made clear, to protect the police from accusations that might arise when dealing with the mentally disordered. The police surgeon provided the police with a medical assessment; that the assessment was not needed in straightforward Section 136 cases is not the point. Nor were the police surgeon's examinations anything more than perfunctory, the usual examination lasting about 5 minutes, and the assessment was almost always 'fit to be detained, fit to be interviewed'. It was an assessment of mental capacity rather than of mental disorder; yet it provided professional advice which was rarely rejected.

Police practices vary, and those which occurred in the East Midlands may not be typical; though if they are, and we suspect they extend to many other police forces, the implications are profound. In this system the police surgeon becomes the genesis of mentally disordered offenders in the criminal justice system because he or she operates at the point where mentally disordered offenders are first seen in the system. These apparently unimportant figures, almost wholly neglected in the research literature, may well turn out to be the key: they determine outcomes by influencing the implementation of Section 136 for non-offender patients and for offenders. Accusations against the police about their failure to identify mentally disordered suspects may turn out to be misplaced; they should be more directed at the police surgeon.

Arrangements for treatment and care

The second part of Section 136 provides for the patient to be detained in a place of safety not exceeding 72 hours, for the purpose of enabling him or her to be examined by a registered medical practitioner and interviewed by an ASW. The role of the ASW was set out in the Butler Committee Report and has changed little since. It includes contacting the detained person's relatives, and ascertaining whether there is a history of psychiatric treatment. Should admission to hospital prove necessary, this information may indicate which hospital would be most suitable; but the ASW should always consider whether any course other than hospital is appropriate. Knowing the range of resources which is available the approved social worker is in a position to assess all the circumstances and is responsible for making sure whether treatment in hospital is the only solution. (Home Office 1975: para. 9.1)

Almost all the literature on Section 136 comments on the need to establish agreed policies and to promote liaison between the police and the health and social services. Practices vary (Home Office 1990: para. 4(I)) and not always to the patient's advantage. The police complain about delays caused by ASWs, ASWs complain about the lack of cooperation with the psychiatrists, and the psychiatrists just complain. Introducing and operating a system where three agencies work together is never going to be easy; agency cooperation within the criminal justice system is rarely achieved. Had the Government accepted some of the recommendations put in the Committee stage of the Bill leading to the 1983 Act to reduce the assessment period from 72 hours to 6 or 8 hours, perhaps a greater sense of urgency might have been conveyed and cooperation increased. One body has now suggested reducing the time to 12 hours (Royal College of Psychiatrists 1997), but this is still too long. As things stand, some ASWs may think there is no need to rush. Paragraph 3.10 of the PACE Code of Practice states:

it is imperative that a mentally disordered or mentally handicapped person who has been detained under Section 136 of the Mental Health Act 1983 should be assessed as soon as possible. If that assessment takes place at a police station by an ASW then a registered medical practitioner should be called to the police station as soon as possible in order to interview that person.

(quoted in Jones 1991)

The Mental Health Act Commission says that 'ASWs need to be available to respond at any hour to calls for Section 136 assessment' (Mental Health Act Commission 1993: 45). The Reed Report (Department of Health/Home Office 1992: para. 11.164) requested that services for mentally disordered offenders be part of local authorities' care plan. The financial and training requirements in the Reed Report need not concern us here, although without a clear set of agreements about who pays for the services, Section 136 will not operate effectively. In the case of patients not admitted to hospital after assessment has taken place, Trusts have been urged to establish systematic procedures to provide for them (Mental Health Act Commission 1993: 45).

Why does this part of Section 136 create such difficulties, and how could the level of complaints be reduced? Part of the answer lies in the drafting of the legislation, a strong hint to future legislators that a new Mental Health Act should clarify that agencies concerned have an obligation to provide the service, i.e. ASWs and psychiatrists should be required to make the necessary arrangements when called to a place of safety. Another lies in the development of a clear operational policy on how Section 136 is to be implemented. There are important regional variations; London differs from elsewhere, while, for example, the Nottingham police have long had an agreement with the local psychiatric services for psychiatrists to attend police stations when called. This rarely happens elsewhere, and in London patients are taken long distances to the mental hospitals responsible for their catchment areas. None the less, policies need to be agreed and acted upon. The Royal College of Psychiatrists sets out detailed procedures and argues that it is reasonable to expect a suitable Responsible Medical Officer and an ASW to attend a place of safety to make an assessment within one hour of being requested to do so. It recognises these are 'stringent' expectations, but 'justified by the seriousness of the situation inherent in the use of Section 136' (Royal College of Psychiatrists 1997: 14). Were that to be followed, and were there to be a standard set of documents to include patients transferred from the police to the hospital, many difficulties would be eased.

Future developments

It is sometimes difficult to believe that when the 1983 Mental Health Act was debated, the decarceration movement had hardly begun. In the years following the pace of change has accelerated, and existing legislation has become dated.

Section 136, like much else in the 1983 Act, is beginning to show its age, not in the sense that the terminology needs tightening, though it surely does, nor in the sense that procedures and guidelines need to be introduced – they were required anyway, irrespective of decarceration, but in the sense that changes have occurred which make Section 136 less effective.

The first relates to the AA. There is a growing awareness of the importance of the AA, a requirement of PACE but rarely used except for children (Bean and Nemitz 1993). Home Office Circular 66/90, whose aim was 'to draw the attention of the courts and those services responsible for dealing with mentally disordered persons who commit, or are suspected of committing criminal offences' made no mention of the AA, an omission which is difficult to understand, especially as it was aimed *inter alia* at Chief Officers of Police. The Mental Health Act Commission Report remedies this, stating that an AA should be asked to attend the police station for anyone detained in a police station which is acting as a place of safety under Section 136 (Mental Health Act Commission 1993: 45). New AA voluntary schemes are providing more trained AAs to service an increasing number of police stations.

The second development relates to changes in the nature of the population being served. When the Act was drafted, mental hospitals were still in the ascendancy. Now there are many patients in the community, and many with a serious drug problem, posing seemingly intractable problems. Dual diagnosis is a common broad term indicating the simultaneous presence of two or more independent disorders, normally a psychiatric disorder and a drug problem. Combinations of conditions show great variability, but common examples include major depression with cocaine, poly-drug use with schizophrenia, and borderline personality disorder with episodic drug use. They vary along important dimensions, such as severity, chronicity, disability and degree of impairment (Department of Health and Human Services [US] 1994: 4). The two disorders may be severe or mild, or one may be more severe than the other, and both may change over time.

Dual-diagnosis patients, who may also be addicted to alcohol or be HIV positive, often experience severe problems because they are vulnerable to relapses from both conditions, and a deterioration in one can lead to the worsening of the other. 'Compared with patients who have a single disorder, patients with dual disorders often require longer treatment, have more crises and progress more gradually in treatment' (Department of Health and Human Services [US] 1994: 4). The American experience suggests that the prevalence of dual diagnosis will increase, since patients with mental disorders have an increased risk of drug use, and patients with drug use have an increased risk of mental disorders. About 33 per cent of American patients with a psychiatric disorder also engage in drug abuse, (about twice the expected rate when compared with non-psychiatric populations) and about 60 per cent of those who use and abuse drugs are mentally disordered (ibid.).

The American experience suggests that primary health care workers will continue to be an important first point of contact for dual-diagnosis patients, being able to provide treatment and follow-up information about their condition. There is no reason to suppose the prevalence and incidence of dual diagnosis in Britain to be less than in the USA: rates of mental disorder and drug abuse are similar in the two countries, albeit that the level of decarceration is less in Britain. Accordingly, diagnosis and treatment produce difficulties, since while all diagnoses have to be provisional and constantly evaluated – there is nothing new or wrong with that – what is required is for primary health care workers to be aware of dual conditions and to know that they complicate diagnosis. For example, conditions often mimic each other – heroin addiction can mimic a mood disorder, and acute manic symptoms can be mimicked by stimulants, steroids, hallucinogens or poly-drug combinations. Similar conditions may be caused by withdrawal from depressants such as alcohol, and by medical disorders such as HIV and thyroid problems. And there are specific disorders that can complicate diagnosis of addiction, including schizophrenia, brief reactive psychosis and anxiety disorder (Department of Health and Human Services [US] 1994: 31).

Treatment is no less complicated. For example, caution is advised when prescribing psychoactive mood-altering medication for dual-diagnosis patients, and referrals to appropriate agencies are likely to be more difficult than hitherto. These and other treatment problems are not of direct concern to the police, but because they are the first to meet the patient and to operate a screening process, they have to be aware of them. And without that they will neither look for them nor report them. Moreover, screening for dual disorders may take longer than screening for a single disorder. That means adjusting to a new set of procedures and a new workload.

Conclusions

Enough has been said to show that the police have a key role in dealing with the mentally disordered in a public place. Nor is there likely to be a diminution of that role; if anything, given existing conditions and likely developments in community care, it may increase. What is required is attention to a number of features, if that role is to be strengthened and allow the police to function effectively. Two are listed here: legislation and the practices of the police and others.

Changes to legislation will help ease some of the more pressing problems. These changes are needed not just to tidy up existing legislation, but to emphasise the need for greater coordination between the agencies. Specifically, this means defining certain terms such as 'public place' and the time at which a Section 136 Order begins. Reducing the period from 72 hours to 6 hours would inject a greater sense of urgency than exists at present, and clarifying the number of places in which a patient may be detained under a place of safety order would be of value.

It would also help if Governments and others would stop believing and suggesting that a police station was inappropriate as a place of safety, since for some suspects it is the only option, and the only one suitable for those who are violent. The Mental Health Act Commission has began to point the way, saying that what is needed is an agreed policy where it is recognised that the police station must accept certain types of patients, while others should be taken elsewhere. In other words, accept that a range of options, which include the police station, is needed.

So far as changing the way the Section operates is concerned, the most elementary reform would be to introduce a method of formally recording all suspects detained under Section 136. This should be completed by the police at the time of arrest and would provide statistical information about the extent of its use. It might also sharpen up practice if the police knew their decisions were being recorded formally. Yet most of all a formal record would help clarify their duties, so that for example, the police would not continue to call a police surgeon when they should be calling an ASW. Were this to be reinforced by clear directions from the Home Office about the respective duties of police, ASWs, and of course psychiatrists, then so much the better.

The Government wants to reform the Mental Health Act 1983; this means the opportunities are there to make the necessary changes. Herschel Prins is concerned that this group of highly vulnerable people – for these purposes suspects on a Section 136 – are landing up in the penal system (Prins 1993), and he is right to express those fears. Section 136 is more than a section dealing with a few patients detained in a public place, for as pointed out above, it is the route into the penal system for many mentally disordered offenders. If we are to take Herschel Prins' fears seriously, we must take Section 136 seriously too.

Notes

1 Section 136 of the Mental Health Act 1983 states:

> (1) If a constable finds in a place to which the public have access a person who appears to him to be suffering from mental disorder and to be in immediate need of care or control, the constable may, if he thinks it necessary to do so in the interests of that person or for the protection of other persons, remove that person to a place of safety within the meaning of Section 135 above.
> (2) A person removed to a place of safety under this Section may be detained for a period not exceeding 72 hours for the purpose of enabling him to be examined by a registered medical practitioner and to be interviewed by an approved social worker and of making any necessary arrangements for his treatment or care.

2 Alongside Section 136 there is the complementary Section 135 which not only gives the definition of a place of safety. (In this Section 'place of safety' means residential accommodation provided by a local social services authority under Part 111 of the National Assistance Act 1948 or under paragraph 2 of Schedule 8 to the National Health Service Act 1977, a hospital as defined by this Act, a police station, a mental nursing home or residential home for mentally disordered persons or any other suitable place the occupier of which is willing temporarily to receive the patient) but provides for a Magistrate to issue a warrant authorising a policeman to enter private premises, using force if necessary, for the purpose of removing a mentally disordered person. Jones (1991) cites the Police and Criminal Evidence Act 1984, Section 17(1)(e) which

says a policeman may enter and search any premises without obtaining a warrant under this Section if such action is required to save 'life or limb' or to prevent 'serious damage to property'. The police also have power to enter premises without a search warrant for the purpose of 'recapturing a person who is unlawfully at large and who is pursuing' (Section 17(1)9a). No research seems to have been done on the operation of these sections.

References

Bean, P.T. (1980) *Compulsory Admissions to Mental Hospitals*. Chichester: John Wiley.
Bean, P.T. *et al.* (1991) *Out of Harm's Way*. London: MIND Publications.
Bean, P.T. and Nemitz, T. (1993) 'Out of depth and out of sight'. Report to MENCAP on the Implementation of the Appropriate Adult Scheme. Unpublished mimeograph.
Bluglass, R. (1984) *A Guide to the Mental Health Act 1983*. London: Churchill Livingstone.
Bynoe, I. (1993) 'The role of the criminal justice agencies in the diversion of mentally disordered offender'. In Mental Health Foundation 'Diversion, care and justice'. (Pre-conference briefing pack).
Department of Health (1997) *Statistical Bulletin: In-patients formally Detained in Hospitals under the Mental Health Act 1983 and Other Legislation, England 1990–91 to 1995–6*. London: HMSO.
Department of Health and Human Services (US) (1994) *Assessment and Treatment of Patients with Coexisting Mental Illness and Alcohol and other Drug Abuse*. Washington, DC: US Government Printing Office.
Department of Health/Home Office (1992) *Review of Health and Social Services for Mentally Disordered Offenders and Others Requiring Similar Services*. (Chairman John Reed). Final Summary Report Cm. 2088. London: HMSO.
Department of Health and Social Security (1976) *A Review of the Mental Health Act 1959*. Consultation Document. Cmnd. 7320. London: HMSO.
Hoggett, B. (1984) *Mental Health Law*. 2nd edition. London: Sweet and Maxwell.
Home Office (1975) *Report of the Committee on Mentally Abnormal Offenders*. (The Butler Report). Cmnd 6144. London: HMSO.
—— (1990) *Provision for Mentally Disordered Offenders*. Home Office Circular no. 66/90. London: Home Office.
Jones, R. (1991) *Mental Health Act Manual*. 3rd edition. London: Sweet and Maxwell.
Mental Health Act Commission (1993) *Fifth Biennial Report 1991–1993*. London: HMSO.
National Association for the Care and Resettlement of Offenders (1993) *Diverting Mentally Disturbed Offenders from Prosecution*. Report of the NACRO Mental Health Advisory Committee. London: NACRO.
Nemitz, T. (1997) 'The use of the appropriate adult for mentally disordered suspects in the police station.' Unpublished PhD thesis. Loughborough: Loughborough University.
Prins, H. (1993) 'Offending patients: the people nobody owns'. In W. Watson and A. Grounds (eds) *The Mentally Disordered Offender in an Era of Community Care*. Cambridge: Cambridge University Press.
Rassaby, E. and Rogers, A. (1987) 'Psychiatric referrals from the police: variations in disposal at different places of safety'. *Bulletin of the Royal College of Psychiatrists*. 11, 78–81.

Rogers, A. (1993) 'Police and psychiatrists: a case of professional dominance'. *Social Policy and Administration*. 27, 33–44.

Rogers, A. and Faulkner, A. (1987) *A Place of Safety*. London: MIND Publications.

Royal College of Psychiatrists (1997) *Standards of Places of Safety under Section 136 of the Mental Health Act 1983*. Council Report CR61. London: RCP.

Taylor, P. T. *et al.* (1993) 'The mentally disordered offender in non-medical settings'. In J. Gunn and P.J. Taylor (eds) *Forensic Psychiatry: Clinical, Legal, and Ethical issues*. London: Butterworth-Heinemann.

Chapter 4

Diverting mentally disordered offenders from custody

Paul Cavadino

For a variety of reasons – part fiscal, part genuinely reformist – the 1990s have seen increasing attention being paid by policy-makers, practitioners and researchers to the plight of mentally disordered people detained in the prison system. A number of studies have been carried out to assess the scale and nature of the problem and a range of initiatives have been undertaken with the aim of diverting mentally disordered offenders and defendants from prison service custody. All these reflect in some way or another the concern with how best to 'manage' the mentally disordered offender, though the particular emphasis here is on the way in which care and treatment are balanced with the workings of the criminal justice system.

This chapter summarises the available research findings and describes the initiatives so far taken to address this issue. It concludes by considering what further action is now needed to ensure that mentally disordered people caught up in the criminal justice process receive the care and treatment which they need in their own and society's best interests.

How many mentally disordered prisoners are there?

A survey of sentenced prisoners carried out by John Gunn and his colleagues for the Home Office and published in 1991 estimated the prevalence of psychiatric disorders among sentenced prisoners at 38.8 per cent (of which disorders related to substance dependency or abuse accounted for 19.6 per cent). They estimated that 3 per cent of the sentenced prison population (approximately 1,100 prisoners) were suffering from psychiatric disorders warranting transfer to an NHS hospital. The findings of the study, which were based on a sample of 5 per cent of prisoners serving sentences of six months or more, are summarised in Table 4.1.

An even higher proportion of prisoners on remand have mental health problems. A recent research study of 750 male remand prisoners in thirteen adult prisons and three young offender institutions (Brooke *et al.* 1996) found that a psychiatric disorder (again widely defined to include substance misuse) was present in 63 per cent of inmates. Apart from substance misuse, which was

Table 4.1 Psychiatric disorders among sentenced prisoners

Diagnosis	Number	Percentage
Psychosis	724	1.9
Neurotic disorders	2,015	5.3
Personality disorders	3,096	8.2
Sexual deviations	710	1.7
Substance abuse/dependence	7,427	19.6
Organic disorders	331	0.9
Uncertain	437	1.2
Total	14,740	38.8

diagnosed in 38 per cent of cases, the main diagnoses were for neurotic illness (26 per cent); personality disorder (11 per cent); and psychosis (5 per cent). The researchers judged that 9 per cent of the sample needed transfer to an NHS hospital. Extrapolation of these results suggested that the remand population as a whole contained 680 men who needed transfer to hospital for psychiatric treatment.

In their commentary on these findings the authors note that:

> it is government policy that prisoners on remand who have a serious mental disorder should be transferred to a psychiatric hospital but this is often not done. Even when a prisoner is transferred there are delays, during which the patient remains in prison and is at increased risk or self-harm and suicide.

They go on to conclude that:

> In addition to causing unnecessary suffering to mentally ill prisoners, this situation creates a risk to the public. Three recent inquiries into killing by mentally ill people described previous remands in custody, during which mental disorder was recognised but not adequately managed. Some of the most difficult psychiatric patients in the country are assessed and treated entirely within prisons, which are not designed for this purpose and cannot match the standards of hospitals.
>
> (Brooke *et al.* 1996: 18–22)

The impact of custody

Defendants who are suspected of being mentally disordered are often remanded in custody for medical reports: there were 2,481 such remands in the year ending 31 March 1995. Yet prison is the worst possible place for someone with a mental disorder. The gloomy conditions inside large Victorian prisons, together with restricted regimes which mean that mentally disturbed prisoners may be locked in their cells for much of the day, are likely to exacerbate the mental health problems of prisoners prone to depression and those who have a disorder with a depressive element.

There is a measure of 'official' recognition of this. The Chief Inspector of Prisons commented in his annual report for 1995–96 as follows:

> We are concerned in particular about the number of prisoners with mental health problems, whose condition prison is more likely to worsen than improve . . . it has to be said that, although many health care staff in prisons can demonstrate an ever wider range of qualifications and flexibility in their work and working practices, the overall service provided across all establishments does not match up to National Health Service standards . . . unless proper care is provided, prison can exacerbate mental health problems, which has a long-term impact on the individual concerned and the community into which he or she may be released.
>
> (1996: 22–23)

Echoing this broader policy dimension is the vivid description by one prison doctor of what it is like to 'reside' and work within such a setting:

> I unlock the door to the ward each morning and experience the same mixture of emotions and feelings as I did on the first day – disgust, despair and nausea. I try to walk about 20 metres which will take me to the relative sanctuary of my office. In doing so I pass several cells. Out of some the prisoners watch me and into some I peer . . . In the first cell there is a naked and contorted body lying on the floor next to a torn mattress; faeces are dumped on the wall and food lies under foot. From the next a face appears at the hatch, 'Hey Doc, when are you going to get me out of here?' I avoid his eye contact, knowing that all our conversations end in threatened violence. In the next a man in strip conditions paces, mumbling to himself and occasionally shouting at his private demons . . .
>
> This . . . represents my own experience of working as a psychiatrist in a prison hospital. Actually, that is not entirely true and therein lies the problem – it is not a hospital, it is a prison health centre. Prisoners cannot be treated against their will in the prison system, except urgent treatment given under common law. That crucial difference denies insightless psychotic men the opportunity of treatment, even when they have been found guilty of an offence, even when the diagnosis is not in doubt, and even when they are waiting transfer to hospital.
>
> (Needham-Bennett and Cumming 1995: 516)

Such conditions can increase the risk of suicide or self-mutilation. In the research carried out by Dooley (1990), the records of prison suicide in England and Wales between 1972 and 1987 were examined. He found that:

- mental disorder was among the reasons for suicide in 22 per cent of cases;
- over a third of prisoners committing suicide had a previous history of psychiatric contact and over a quarter had previous in-patient admission;
- 23 per cent had received some form of psychotropic medication in the month before suicide.

Later studies support the connections between mental disturbance and either suicide or various forms of self-harm. For example, Liebling and Krarup's study (1993) of suicide attempts and self-injury at 16 prisons found that 34 per cent of the sample had been receiving medical or psychiatric treatment at the time of the incident, and of the 60 self-inflicted deaths in prison in 1995-96, the Prison Service Director of Health Care reported that 28 (47 per cent) had a known previous psychiatric history (HM Prison Service 1997).

The remand process

An earlier study of mentally disordered remand prisoners (Grounds *et al.* 1991) was carried out for the Home Office. The study recorded details of all men and women remanded in custody to Holloway, Brixton and Risley prisons over a 5- to 6-month period during 1989 who came to the attention of prison doctors for psychiatric reasons. The group comprised 952 cases in all (698 men and 254 women).

Only a small proportion had been charged with serious crimes of violence. Most had been charged with relatively minor offences: thefts, public nuisance offences and criminal damage predominated. A substantial proportion (40 per cent in London) had no proper home and had been living in unsettled accommodation, or on the streets. Not surprisingly, the authors concluded that homelessness was clearly an important factor in decisions to remand such defendants in custody.

Over half the sample (507 of 952) were thought by prison doctors to be suffering from psychiatric illness. For the majority of this group (76 per cent in Brixton, 66 per cent in Risley and 85 per cent in Holloway), the prison doctors made referrals to outside psychiatrists, in the hope that an assessment visit would be followed by the offer of a hospital bed. Once referrals were made, the prison doctors usually wrote to the courts requesting remands to allow time for these visits to take place, and these requests were generally granted.

In the summary of the research which appeared in 1992, the authors commented that 'the first effect of a referral to an outside psychiatrist is therefore substantially to lengthen the time that a mentally ill person spends in prison'. They continue – pointing to the paradox that efforts to secure the most appropriate health care causes questionable extensions in imprisonment for those who have yet to be tried for their offences:

> Psychiatrists who work in the community have different perspectives from those working in prison, and when they agreed about the nature and

degree of the prisoner's illness, they were liable to disagree about whether hospitalisation was necessary . . . It would often have been appropriate on psychiatric grounds to seek a further opinion about placement, for example from a regional forensic psychiatrist, but seeking a further opinion for remand prisoners means seeking further time in custody. Prison doctors are thus in the intolerable position of being able to pursue appropriate care for their patients only at the cost of imposing additional terms of imprisonment on them.

(Grounds *et al.* 1992: 2–3)

In Holloway, for example, the average remand time in custody for psychotic women referred only to one consultant was 28 days, whereas for those referred to more than one it was 63 days. Delays in assessments by outside psychiatrists – not only for these prisoners in Holloway, but for all remand prisoners – are aggravated by the difficulties which consultants often face in obtaining access to prisoners. These can include:

- long waits in being escorted from the prison gate to the health care centre and before the prisoner is brought to the psychiatrist;
- the inflexibility of prison regimes which can prevent appointments being made at the beginning or end of the working day, or at lunchtimes and week-ends, thus requiring a consultant to cancel an out-patient clinic in order to assess perhaps one prisoner;
- the prison environment itself, which may not be conducive to carrying out a psychiatric assessment because of, for example, the size, availability and position of rooms;
- the long distances from their home areas at which some prisoners are held when they have offended in another area or are transferred because of prison overcrowding.

The researchers found that when visiting doctors offered to provide beds, it was nearly always under a hospital order made under Section 37 of the Mental Health Act 1983. Even after the orders were made, the subjects were routinely sent back to prison to await admission for up to the 28 days which the Act permits. Yet, had the same people been seen by the same psychiatrists in the community they would, under civil procedures, have been admitted to hospital within 24 hours. In drawing together the implications of their research, Grounds and his colleagues concluded that:

Although there was variation in the medical organisation and practice of the three establishments . . . all were totally unsuitable places in terms of regime and physical conditions in which to house mentally disordered people. Why then should all these people, so few of whom were thought to require imprisonment when sentenced, have been sent to prison on remand? It seemed clear . . . that this was not because of the seriousness of their offences, but because of their apparent need for help: the courts were using remand prisons as social and psychiatric assessment and referral centres . . . [R]emands in custody [are] not only an inhumane, but [are] an ineffective way of securing help and care for disturbed people. For those who obtained hospital places it meant weeks or months of imprisonment, at the end of which they were admitted to beds for which they had been qualified at the outset. And for the mentally ill people who were not offered beds, the process was equally unsatisfactory. In most cases they were petty offenders without social roots, for whom magistrates had evidently ordered custodial remands in the hope that some kind of solution to their problems would be found. After weeks in prison they were generally discharged back to the situations they had come from without the courts being able to arrange for accommodation, treatment or support . . . [A]s a method of obtaining psychiatric help for mentally disordered offenders, the custodial remand has nothing to commend it . . . [I]t exposes mentally disordered people to conditions and regimes which are cruelly harsh and inappropriate. It brings into prison thousands of defendants who do not need to be there and for whom penal disposals are never contemplated.

(Grounds *et al.* 1992: 4–6)

'Bailable' remand prisoners

Kennedy *et al.* (1997) examined the number and characteristics of mentally vulnerable defendants who appeared before the main Inner London magistrates' courts between April and September 1993. The researchers identified 495 cases in which there was clear evidence that the defendant had a mental health problem, 312 of whom were remanded in custody. They found that there was a highly significant difference in the proportions bailed, depending on housing status: 83.6 per cent of those with stable housing were granted bail, compared with 46.6 per cent of those without. Some 10 per cent of those remanded in custody received prison sentences of between two and ten months.

The researchers identified 105 cases, or an estimated annual total of 230, whom they considered to be potentially ' bailable', that is whose current office was not serious and who had no serious previous offences. This group were mostly male, in their early thirties, poorly housed and often with an unclear or changing mental health diagnosis. Drawing out the implications of their data, the authors note that:

They had all been remanded in custody, often because of concern about their lack of housing and ability to return to court. It would seem that even in those cases where bail was granted, without the necessary housing and support people are very likely to 'fail bail' and therefore face an increased risk of being remanded on custody at their next court appearance. Why was this group of people held in custody on remand when so few actually went to prison at the end of the court process?

Based on an estimated six weeks average length of stay by bail cases in probation hostels, this 'bailable' group would require twenty-five to thirty permanent bedspaces which might be provided by specialised units or psychiatric support to existing hostels. The researchers concluded with the following proposal:

> we have found evidence that there is a substantial group, about 20% of all mental health cases in inner London magistrates' courts, who might benefit from some form of psychiatric bail provision as an alternative to custody. This group is characterised by lack of housing, non-serious offences, and indeterminate psychiatric diagnosis. They appear to pose an insufficient risk of 'dangerousness' to justify the costly and damaging aspects of remands in custody.
>
> (Kennedy *et al.* 1997: 167)

Black defendants

One study (NACRO 1990) of seventy cases in which a magistrates' court asked for psychiatric reports on defendants, found that black defendants were less likely than white defendants to be granted bail and that lengths of custodial remands were greater for black defendants. The court was in an area with a black population of between 15 and 20 per cent. Of the seventy defendants in the sample, 33 per cent were black, 39 per cent were white, 2 per cent Asian and in 26 per cent of cases the defendant's race was not clear from court records. Some 37 per cent of the white defendants were granted bail compared with 13 per cent of black defendants, a difference which could only partly be accounted for by the number of previous convictions or the seriousness of the offences charged. The report observed that 'decision makers seemed more likely to err on the side of caution with black mentally vulnerable defendants and to be affected by a heightened perception of dangerousness with regard to this group' (ibid.: 35).

Diversion from custody

Home Office Circular 66/90, *Provision for Mentally Disturbed Offenders*, said that 'a mentally disordered person should never be remanded to prison simply to receive medical treatment or assessment' and that 'it is government policy that, wherever possible, mentally disordered persons should receive care and treatment from the health and social services'. Subsequent official guidance, issued in 1995, reiterated this: 'The Government supports the policy that mentally disordered people who require treatment and support because of their health care needs should be cared for or treated . . . as far as possible, in the community rather than in institutional settings' (Home Office and Department of Health 1995: 12).

There are potentially many routes for diverting mentally disturbed people into psychiatric care. If the police suspect mental disorder in someone behaving in a disturbed manner in a public place, under Section 136 of the Mental Health Act 1983 they can remove the person to a place of safety which may be a police station, a hospital or any other setting considered appropriate, where he or she must be assessed by a registered medical practitioner and an approved social worker. Assessments might lead to diversion to a psychiatric hospital under a civil section of the Mental Health Act or admission on an informal basis. Alternatively, the person may be referred to a community health service or agency. If someone has been arrested for an alleged criminal offence, the police are required to arrange for a professional assessment by a registered medical practitioner if the person appears to be mentally disordered. Here again, assessment may lead to admission to hospital under a civil section of the Mental Health Act or on an informal basis (whether or not prosecution is pursued).

Where the person is detained overnight in the police station, in many areas they will be interviewed by a bail information officer working for a probation service bail information scheme. If it becomes apparent that the offender is mentally disordered, information can be passed to the Crown Prosecution Service. The probation service can also alert the court to the possibility the defendant is mentally disturbed, as may a solicitor representing him or her. This may lead to assessment and reports, which can result in arrangements for support and treatment.

The Crown Prosecution Service may decide, in the light of information about the person's mental condition, that prosecution would not be in the public interest. If the person is proceeded against and appears in court, the courts have powers to remand to hospital for assessment or for treatment under, respectively, Sections 35 and 36 of the Mental Health Act 1983. Under Section 48 of the Mental Health Act, prisoners on remand can be transferred to hospital provided that the person is suffering from a mental disorder 'of a nature or degree which makes it appropriate for him to be detained in a hospital for treatment and . . . such treatment is likely to alleviate or prevent a deterioration of his condition'. Section 47 of the Act, which contains a similar power in relation to sentenced prisoners, and Section 48 were used between them in 746 cases in 1996. There has been a significant and welcome increase in the number transferred in recent years: in 1983 the total was 94.

At the sentencing stage, Section 3 of the Criminal Justice Act 1991 requires courts to obtain a pre-sentence report when they are considering a custodial sentence, unless they consider that this would be unnecessary. These reports, prepared by the probation service, may include reference to any concern about the offender's mental health. Under Section 4 of the Act, courts are required to obtain a medical report before passing a custodial sentence on an offender who is or appears to be mentally disordered. Courts' sentencing options include making probation orders with psychiatric requirements, hospital orders (which can be accompanied by a restriction order in the Crown Court), interim hospital orders and guardianship orders.

Court assessment schemes

In the early 1990s particular attention was given to the role of court psychiatric assessment schemes in diverting mentally disordered defendants from custody. Home Office Circular 66/90 commended the court psychiatric assessment arrangements which were then in operation at Peterborough and certain central London magistrates' courts. It said:

> These enable the courts to receive speedy medical advice and to ensure that, where appropriate, arrangements can be made quickly to admit a mentally disordered person to hospital, for example, as a condition of bail, or with the agreement of the hospital managers, under Section 35 of the Mental Health Act 1983 following conviction.
>
> (Home Office 1990: para.7)

A study of a psychiatric liaison service at Clerkenwell Magistrates' Court (James and Hamilton 1991), illustrated the benefits of such a service. This was established between the Department of Psychiatry at the Royal Free Hospital and Clerkenwell and Hampstead Magistrates' Courts, sitting at Clerkenwell. Two psychiatrists (the authors of the article) attended court one day a week to examine people in custody for whom psychiatric reports had been requested. Those appearing in court on days when the psychiatrists were not present were remanded until the day of the psychiatrists' next visit.

The psychiatrists examined those referred in the cell area and gave oral reports to the court on the same day. Recommendations were completed for hospital admissions under both Part II (the civil sections) and Part III (the court sections) of the Mental Health Act 1983. Where hospital orders were made, direct admission to hospital from the court was arranged if possible. The authors compared the outcomes of 80 referrals to the psychiatric liaison scheme over a 9-month period with those of 50 consecutive cases contemporaneously placed on hospital orders by London magistrates' courts after being remanded to Brixton prison for the preparation of reports. For the latter, the mean time from arrest to hospital admission was 50.8 days. Of the 80 referrals to the Clerkenwell psychiatric liaison scheme, the psychiatrists recommended hospital admissions in 39 cases: the courts accepted the recommendations in all these instances. Of the 39 hospital orders made, 25 (64 per cent) were under Part II (the civil sections) of the Act. For those reaching hospital through the scheme, the mean number of days from arrest to admission was 8.7 days. This was accomplished because the scheme virtually abolished three of the waiting periods: those from the request to assessment, from assessment to the order being made, and from the order being made to admission to hospital. For those assessed under the liaison scheme but not sent to hospital, the mean time from arrest to appearance in court with a report was 5.4 days, compared with 33.7 days for those assessed in prison.

Following the introduction of the psychiatric liaison scheme, Clerkenwell Court made an average of 4.3 hospital orders a month – a rate four times that for the previous twelve months, after adjusting for a 9 per cent increase in those appearing before the court between the two periods. In the light of their evidence, the authors concluded:

> The psychiatric liaison scheme to the magistrates' court resulted in a con-siderable decrease in the number of days that those remanded for psychiatric reports spent in custody compared with the traditional practice of obtaining second opinions at the remand prison. This reduction was greater than 80%, both for those sent to hospital and those not. For those placed on hospital orders the scheme achieved this reduction both by accelerating the provision of a report to a court and by arranging admission to a hospital on the day the order was made.
>
> (James and Hamilton 1991: 284)

A study of another psychiatric assessment scheme (Joseph and Potter 1993a) based at Bow Street and Marlborough Street magistrates' court also points to the benefits that can arise from effective inter-agency communication and co-ordination. A psychiatrist was available on the same two mornings each week: on other days defendants were remanded in custody until the next day on which the psychiatrist visited. The referral criterion was 'those defendants perceived by any court official as requiring a psychiatric assessment who might be, or had already been, remanded into custody for a medical report'. The psychiatrist gave oral evidence in court consisting of an opinion regarding fitness to plead, the diagnosis if any, and a medical recommendation. To facilitate hospital admission under the civil provisions of the Mental Health Act 1983, the approved social worker from the local social services department attended court if hospital admission was indicated, and a second psychiatrist was also available.

Over the eighteen months of the study, 201 referrals were made to the service, 101 from Bow Street and 100 from Marlborough Street. Some individuals were referred more than once, and the sample consisted of 185 people. The majority of people referred were of no fixed abode and socially isolated. At the time of their arrest 68 (37 per cent) were living on the streets and a further 52 (28 per cent)

Table 4.2 Diagnoses of referrals

Diagnosis	Number	Percentage
Schizophrenia	72	39
Manic-depressive psychosis	21	11
Other psychoses	18	10
Neurosis/personality disorder	28	15
Alcohol/drug dependence	20	11
Mental retardation	4	2
Uncertain/no diagnosis	22	12
Total	185	100

were living in unsettled accommodation, namely night shelters, hostels, bed and breakfasts or squats. Only one-third (65) were living in stable accommodation and altogether three-quarters were living alone; 163 (88 per cent) were unemployed, the majority for over a year. They were predominantly petty offenders with numerous convictions: theft was the most common previous office with assault, criminal damage and public order offences also represented. The primary diagnoses for the 185 defendants were shown in Table 4.2 on p. 62.

Following initial assessment, 51 (25 per cent) were admitted directly to hospital, 101 (50 per cent) were released, and 49 (24 per cent) were returned to custody. Of the 51 hospital admissions, 44 were admitted on the day of assessment and a further 7 within a few days.

A further 14 defendants were subsequently admitted to hospital via custody, making a total of 65 hospital admissions. For those admitted directly to hospital, the average time from court to admission was 5.8 days; the 14 custody cases took an average of 35 days; for all 65 hospital admissions the average time was 10 days. The court followed 90 per cent of the scheme's psychiatric recommendations. Some 58 cases (29 per cent) were discontinued by the Crown Prosecution Service: of these, 35 were admitted to hospital and the remainder were released. A further 99 cases (49 per cent) were dealt with non-custodially by conditional discharges, fines or probation orders. In 24 cases (12 per cent) the court made a hospital order under Section 37 of the Mental Health Act. The authors stress what they see as the beneficial outcome of the scheme:

> The psychiatrist in court has access to the CPS or court files, which contain details of the charge, witnesses' statements, and previous convictions, information which is often unavailable to the prison doctor. Furthermore the court probation officer can often provide background information and discuss issues regarding entering a plea. In short, many of the barriers to communication which occur in prison are removed. The opportunity for the psychiatrist to discuss the case with CPS with a view to discontinuance is vital . . . It is virtually unknown for psychiatrists at a prison to recommend the discontinuance of a case on the grounds of public interest.
>
> (Joseph and Potter 1993a: 329)

A follow-up study of the 65 people who were admitted to hospital as a result of the scheme (Joseph and Potter 1993b) found that 50 (77 per cent) derived some or marked benefit from psychiatric treatment. In the three years before the introduction of the service, there was an average of 33 hospital orders per year from the two courts. During the 18 months of the study, there was a total of 81 hospital admissions, including 16 defendants who were not referred to the court psychiatrist – an average of 54 per year. This represented a 64 per cent increase.

Although the most detailed published research studies are of schemes in which psychiatrists attend court, the majority of court assessment schemes use other approaches. Burney and Pearson (1995) evaluated a different model employed by the Islington Mentally Disordered Offenders Project, which was established in April 1992 at Highbury Grove Magistrates' Court. The project employed a psychiatric nurse as a full-time mental health court worker with a remit to assess offenders with possible mental disorders, to assist the court in dealing with them appropriately, and to offer support and training to probation staff. In the first twelve months, the worker processed 101 referrals, 85 of whom she assessed as mentally disordered.

Some were deemed sufficiently ill to justify referral to the Clerkenwell Court's psychiatric assessment scheme. Some were repeated petty offenders who were not so ill as to require immediate hospitalisation: in these instances the mental health court worker provided a link with appropriate support services and in some cases obtained the required health service intervention where the court would have no power to order it. Others reflected the spectrum of mental illness and distress while not suffering from the more obviously recognised psychoses: depression was the most familiar of these conditions. Many such offenders found their way on to probation caseloads where the mental health support worker could be called upon in her support role, enabling probation officers to feel more confident in dealing with such offenders. The researchers commented:

> In the first year of the mental health court worker scheme, information on accommodation was not routinely recorded. However, of the 57 cases where information was held, approximately one-half were living in permanent accommodation, with one-quarter of no fixed abode, and the remainder in some form of temporary accommodation. Even so, individual casework revealed that some of the accommodation described as 'permanent' could be most precarious. Some of the referrals requiring most support are psychotic individuals living without electricity or hot water because of unpaid bills, and with virtually no furniture. One man in such a position had received no help from social services for over a year in spite of requests from the mental health court worker. It was only her intervention that enabled him to receive a disability allowance, and cases such as this point to the potential fragility of 'community care' arrangements . . . This combination of circumstances underlines not only the importance of stable accommodation for mentally disordered people, but also that support of the right kind should be available to minimise the behaviour which can undermine that stability where it might already exist.
>
> (Burney and Pearson 1995: 301)

Another approach, first developed in Hertfordshire, involves a multi-agency assessment panel which coordinates the contributions of various agencies involved in preparing reports on an accused person's mental state and the availability of hospital accommodation or community care. The court thereby receives a more detailed assessment of the accused and information about the available options other than a custodial sentence. A typical panel may include a consultant psychiatrist, a clinical psychologist, a community psychiatric nurse, a probation officer and a social worker. It may also include a general practitioner, a housing officer, an employer and members of the individual's family. The aims of the panel are to encourage closer inter-agency work; to provide courts with more constructive and coherent reports in terms of the assessment of the individual; and to propose a coordinated package which may, where appropriate, include a probation order with or without a condition of psychiatric treatment and which may also involve links with the education and housing services. A Home Office evaluation has concluded that where panel schemes have been operating, they have made a significant contribution to ensuring that properly informed decisions are made about mentally disordered offenders (Hedderman 1993). The fact that staff from several agencies are involved and that there is a real commitment to offer a service means that courts can made decisions with confidence.

A national survey of arrangements in magistrates' courts for diversion from custody (Blumenthal and Wessely, 1992) identified 48 psychiatric assessment schemes, with another 31 under development. These included a variety of arrangements, involving: a full inter-disciplinary team of two psychiatrists; an approved social worker and a community psychiatric nurse; a psychiatrist alone; screening by a community psychiatric nurse, approved social worker or probation officer, with referral to others for action; a multi-disciplinary 'panel' convened upon referral; and schemes where a psychiatrist is on call if required. From April 1993, the Home Office made available funding to meet the sessional costs or fees of psychiatrists or community psychiatric nurses attending magistrates' courts. In 1996, it provided funding for 53 such schemes (Home Office 1997: 25).

Diversion at the police custody stage

A number of areas have developed arrangements to divert mentally disordered people from the penal system by intervention at the police custody stage. For example, the North Humberside Diversion Project consists of a team comprising a probation officer, an approved social worker and two community psychiatric nurses. The team assesses persons in police custody as well as at court, in co-operation with a rota of psychiatrists, and arranges appropriate care including, for example, psychiatric outpatient care, appropriate housing and bail support. A recent evaluation by the University of Hull showed an 85 per cent success rate in diverting mentally disordered offenders from custody, and a re-offending rate of only 12 per cent in the first year of operation (Staite et al. 1994).

A joint guidance document on inter-agency working with mentally disordered offenders, published by the Home Office and the Department of Health in 1995, cited three examples of schemes working at the police custody stage. First, the Barnet Crisis Intervention Service is a 24-hour, 7-days-a-week on-call service in which a multi-disciplinary team (doctor, social worker, community psychiatric nurse) provides support to those experiencing mental health or emotional crises.

Referrals usually come from general practitioners but can also come from the police, when the team will not only assess the individual but also provide follow-up treatment.

Second, the Canterbury and Thanet Community Healthcare Trust has established a procedure whereby a police surgeon, having been called out to the police station by the duty officer, calls on the duty psychiatrist and approved social worker to assess individuals at the police station who might then be directed into health or social care as appropriate. The scheme has resulted in a considerable reduction in the number of mentally disordered offenders having to be referred to the court.

Third, under a scheme established in 1992, a community psychiatric nurse is based at Bourneville Lane police station in Birmingham to offer advice and guidance to the police at three local police stations on how to respond to the needs of mentally disordered offenders, and to obtain access to appropriate psychiatric and social services. The main benefits of the scheme include better and more comprehensive assessments at the police station, improved access to psychiatric services, and the opportunity for the community psychiatric nurse to liaise with other agencies where hospital admission is not appropriate and to offer follow-up care.

The inter-agency approach

The Home Office and the Mental Health Foundation jointly funded three pilot projects undertaken by NACRO from 1990 to 1993 in Birmingham, Kirklees and Liverpool, with the aim of encouraging effective cooperation between those working in the criminal justice system and the health and social services to ensure that the health and care needs of mentally disordered offenders were met.

A key finding from the project was the need for development to be overseen and driven by inter-agency groupings which bring together senior representatives from all the relevant agencies. The evidence from the NACRO projects suggested that where such a body was established with a clear work programme, a great deal could be achieved within the context of existing staffing resources. Important gaps in existing provision were also identified and led to new initiatives (such as the attachment of a community psychiatric nurse to Bourneville Lane police station in Birmingham, referred to above).

In 1996, NACRO was commissioned by the Home Office to undertake a survey of the current state of inter-agency arrangements for dealing with mentally disordered offenders. This found that most areas had a joint health/social services/ police policy on Section 136 of the Mental Health Act 1983 (although less than half had associated practice guidance and procedures) but that only a third of areas had joint policies and procedures on other aspects of arrangements of dealing with mentally disordered offenders (Home Office 1997).

The total number of diversion schemes identified by the survey was 194. The most common model is a community psychiatric nurse based at a single magistrates' court or a cluster of courts (around two-thirds of all schemes) and other models include those where schemes originated at magistrates' courts have expanded to include arrangements for assessments at police stations. About 20 per cent of the identified schemes are operating at police stations only (including arrangements developed for Section 136 cases). The number of schemes and their geographical coverage are encouraging, although some of the funding arrangements are fragile, for example, dependent on a single local agency (mostly health trusts or district authorities) where there is often no long-term commitment

What should be done?

In 1992, the interdepartmental Reed Committee Report recommended that 'there should be nation-wide provision of properly resourced court assessment and diversion schemes' and that 'purchasers and providers of health and social services must regard the availability of assessment and diversion schemes as part of a standard service' (Department of Health and Home Office 1992a: 14). It also made a number of proposals to bring about more effective arrangements to divert mentally disturbed people from police custody to health and social services care.

The Home Office Circular 12/95, *Mentally Disordered Offenders: Inter-Agency Working* (Home Office and Department of Health 1995), asked chief police officers to develop arrangements for the examination by psychiatrists or other mental health professionals of persons detained in police custody, including cases under Section 136 of the Mental Health Act 1983, and to consider setting up mental health assessment schemes at selected police stations. Chief probation officers were asked, in cooperation with other agencies, to ensure that alternatives to prison custody were available to courts before and after conviction and that other effective courses of action were available where prosecution was not necessary in the public interest; to facilitate access to accommodation in order to avoid prison custody having to be used in default of more appropriate accommodation; and to advise the court on possible options other than imprisonment. Magistrates and judges were asked, when making decisions on remands or imprisonment, 'to bear in mind that custody is inefficient as a means solely to obtain medical reports or to meet treatment needs'. Justice clerks were asked to consider, in consultation with other local services and agencies, developing mental health assessment schemes based at magistrates' courts.

There is a powerful case for the establishment of psychiatric assessment services in every police and court area. However, the comments made by Blumenthal and Wessely in their national survey of 1992 remain as apposite now as then:

> Mentally disordered offenders require facilities for treatment and care once they have been diverted from custody . . . Many of the schemes currently operating have adequate provisions for psychiatric assessment but inadequate

arrangements for follow up treatment and care of the offender once diverted from custody.

(Blumenthal and Wessely 1992: 1325)

Additional facilities are needed for mentally disordered offenders and defendants, ranging from secure hospital places to supportive accommodation in the community. Although many defendants and offenders requiring in-patient care can be accommodated in ordinary psychiatric provision, it is also important that there should also be better access to local intensive care and locked wards. The number of medium secure hospital places has increased in recent years, but more such places are still needed.

Other mentally disturbed offenders need services in the community, including access to supportive accommodation for mentally disordered defendants. This will necessitate improving hostels' ability and confidence to deal with mentally disordered defendants and improving access for those on bail to mainstream accommodation services for people with mental health problems. The Reed Committee's Report recognised the need for additional staffing in agencies dealing with mentally disordered offenders, including additional consultant forensic psychiatrist posts.

Other measures which would help in the process of diverting mentally disordered offenders from custody include:

- The establishment at local level of inter-agency groups to coordinate the planning and development of services for mentally disordered offenders and defendants. These should draw up plans for diversion arrangements at different stages of the criminal justice process and plans for monitoring arrangements.
- Those responsible for purchasing and providing services in the health service and local authorities should be required to assess the need for services for mentally disturbed offenders and defendants and to include these in their purchasing plans. Each purchasing authority or agency should designate a specific postholder with responsibility for purchasing services relevant to mentally disturbed offenders.
- Funding to local authorities for community care provision should be ring fenced, with specific provision for the needs of mentally disturbed offenders.

The development of specialist bail support arrangements for defendants who are or appear to be mentally disordered, involving support and supervision by health or social services agencies and/or the probation service, could give courts more confidence to remand defendants on bail rather than in custody for the preparation of psychiatric reports.

Alongside the development of services and facilities, the Reed Committee proposed that consideration be given to changes in the law. Among the possibilities it identified were to empower hospitals to give treatment if necessary under Section 35 of the Mental Health Act 1983 (which at present permits courts to remand to hospital for assessment only); to enable magistrates' courts to remand for hospital treatment under Section 36, which is currently restricted to Crown Courts; and to remove or restrict courts' powers to remand to prison for the primary purpose of medical assessment. The report of the Committee's Prison Advisory Group explained the reasoning behind the latter proposal as follows:

> There is good research evidence that courts remand the mentally disordered in custody essentially for psychiatric and social reasons rather than for reasons of public safety or seriousness of offence. In principle it is wrong that courts should be able to remand to prison for the primary purpose of medical assessment. This is also an unjustifiable use of the prison system. Moreover, from a practical point of view, achieving the policy aim of diverting the mentally disordered from prison requires not only alternative provision but also a restriction in the powers and incentives which encourage existing bad practice to continue. Most of the mentally disordered entering the remand prison population have been remanded by magistrates' courts for medical reports. Removing this power and ensuring that adequate alternative provision is made by the health and social services would close a doorway by which the mentally disordered enter that population. We accordingly recommend that the appropriate powers in the Bail Act 1976 and Magistrates' Courts Act 1980 should be reviewed with a view to amendment or repeal.
>
> (Department of Health and Home Office 1992b)

A less radical legislative proposal would be to extend to remanded defendants the principle underlying Section 4 of the Criminal Justice Act 1991, which requires courts, before passing a custodial sentence on an offender who is or appears to be mentally disordered, to consider the likely effect of such a sentence on the offender's mental condition. There is no equivalent requirement in relation to bail decisions – yet the impact of a remand in custody can be at least as damaging. A new consideration should be added to the list of considerations in paragraph 9 of Part I of Schedule I to the Bail Act, to which the courts must have regard when making bail decisions, namely: 'the state of the mental health of the defendant and the likely effect upon this of a remand in custody'.

Conclusion

Imprisoning mentally disordered offenders is inhumane. It can worsen some disorders and prevent mentally ill people from receiving the treatment they need in their own and society's interests. In recent years there have been welcome moves in many areas to divert such offenders from custody by intervention at the police custody and court stages. This chapter has referred to many of these. The task now is to extend and consolidate diversion initiatives, to develop the improved range of hospital- and community-based facilities which is needed to increase their effectiveness, and to ensure that the process of diversion is effectively integrated into mainstream services.

References

Blumenthal, S. and Wessely, S. (1992) 'National survey of current arrangements for diversion from custody in England and Wales'. *British Medical Journal* 305, 1322–1325.

Brooke, D., Taylor, C., Gunn, J. and Maden, A. (1996) 'Point prevalence of mental disorder in unconvicted male prisoners in England and Wales'. *British Medical Journal* 313, 18–21.

Burney, E. and Pearson, G. (1995) 'Mentally disordered offenders: finding a focus for diversion'. *Howard Journal* 34. 4, 291–313.

Department of Health and Home Office (1992a) *Review of Mental Health and Social Services for Mentally Disordered Offenders and Others Requiring Similar Services.* (The Reed Committee) London: HMSO.

Department of Health and Home Office (1992b) *Review of Mental Health and Social Services for Mentally Disordered Offenders and Others Requiring Similar Services, Volume 2: Service needs. (Community, Hospital and Prison Reports and Steering Committee Overview).* London: HMSO.

Dooley, E. (1990) 'Prison suicide in England and Wales, 1972–87'. *British Journal of Psychiatry* 156, 40–45.

Grounds, A., Dell, S., James, K. and Robertson, G. (1991) *Mentally Disordered Remanded Prisoners: Report to the Home Office.* Cambridge: Cambridge Institute of Criminology.

Grounds, A., Dell, S. and James, K. and Robertson, G. (1992) *Mentally Disordered Remand Prisoners.* Research Bulletin No. 32. London: Home Office Research.

Gunn, J., Maden, A. and Swinton, M. (1991) *Mentally Disordered Prisoners.* London: Home Office.

Hedderman, C. (1993) *Panel Assessment Schemes for Mentally Disordered Offenders.* Research and Planning Unit Paper No. 76. London: Home Office.

HM Chief Inspector of Prisons (1996) *Annual Report of HM Chief Inspector of Prisons for England and Wales, April 1995– March 1996.* London: HMSO.

HM Prison Service (1997) *Report of the Director of Health Care 1995–1996.* London: Home Office.

Home Office (1990) *Provision for Mentally Disordered Offenders.* Circular 66/90. London: Home Office.

Home Office (1997) *Annual Report 1997.* London: HMSO.

Home Office Mental Health Unit (1997) 'Survey of inter-agency arrangements for mentally disordered offenders'. London, unpublished paper prepared for the Criminal Justice Consultative Committee.

Home Office and Department of Health (1995) *Mentally Disordered Offenders: Inter-Agency Working.* London: Home Office and Department of Health.

James, D. and Hamilton, L. (1991) 'The Clerkenwell Scheme: assessing efficacy and cost of a psychiatric liaison service to a magistrates' court'. *British Medical Journal* 303, 282-285.

Joseph, P. and Potter, M. (1993a) 'Diversion from custody 1: psychiatric assessment at the magistrates' court'. *British Journal of Psychiatry.* 162, 325–330.

—— (1993b) 'Diversion from custody II: effect on hospital and prison resources'. *British Journal of Psychiatry* 162, 330–334.

Kennedy, M., Truman, C., Keyes S. and Cameron, A. (1997) 'Supported bail for mentally vulnerable defendants'. *Howard Journal*. 36 (2), 158–169.

Liebling, A. and Krarup, H. (1993) *Suicide Attempts and Self-Injury Inside Prisons*. London: Home Office.

NACRO, Afro-Caribbean Mental Health Association and Commission for Racial Equality (1990) *Black People, Mental Health and the Courts*. London: NACRO.

Needham-Bennett, H. and Cumming, I. (1995) 'Waiting for a disaster to happen'. *British Medical Journal* 311, 516–516.

Staite, C., Martin, M., Bingham, M. and Daly, R. (1994) *Diversion from Custody for Mentally Disordered Offenders*. Harlow: Longman.

Chapter 5

Recreating mayhem?

Developing understanding for social
work with mentally disordered
people

Michael Preston-Shoot

Unravelling complexities, signposting interventions

Amongst the clearest memories of social work training is the answer given to us
by Herschel Prins when, as students, we asked him to name the most important
social work skill. *Look for the not so obvious*. This encouragement to enquire
widely and to think creatively connects with a systemic commitment to concerned
curiosity (Cecchin 1987) and to a psychodynamic emphasis on the internal supervisory viewpoint (Casement 1985). The former is an inquisitive stance which
challenges everything in the search for new possibilities, delaying action until
varying perspectives have been fully understood, even when pressure is applied
for more immediate action. The latter refers to an observing ego which helps
people to disentangle themselves from the action by viewing complex encounters
and co-evolving interactions from different vantage points. Both are concerned to
prevent premature closure on a single view of reality, and to ensure that practice
becomes part of the solution rather than part of the problem.

The tragedies involving mentally disordered people have stimulated much
media, public and political scrutiny. In turn, this has generated considerable
policy momentum, reflected in the introduction of supervised discharge orders
(Mental Health (Patients in the Community) Act 1995) and supervision registers
(HSG(94)5); guidance on risk assessment and the discharge of mentally disordered
people (LASSL (94)4); the application of the Care Programme Approach to
people with a mental illness (LASSL(90)11), and the requirement (LASSL(95)12)
that any homicide committed by a person involved with specialist mental health
services should be followed by an independent inquiry and published report.

Do these developments reflect lessons learned? Have they followed an
exploration of the complexity which is practice with mentally disordered people,
eschewing simple cause and effect punctuations of reality, or are they a pragmatic
response which reduces complex phenomena to manageable bits and pieces, and
which thereby prescribes solutions before fully defining and understanding the
problem (Preston-Shoot and Agass 1990)? Zito and Howlett (1996) are critical of
mental health service planning and provision, and of the underpinning community

care policy which have emerged from these developments. Describing the situation as dangerous, they point to demoralised professionals working in difficult conditions; to unfocused services lacking the basic requirements of training, finance, supervision and planning; and to people left to deteriorate in situations which increase their vulnerability and the risk of harm.

They are not alone in describing as a disaster the policy of caring for mentally ill people in the community. The Commission on Social Justice (1994) referred to care in the community as a failing policy, characterised by inadequate resources and people being passed between agencies at the expense of appropriate forms of care. A Mental Health Foundation inquiry (Faulkner 1994) concluded that government policy was undermining community care, arguing that it was deeply flawed, confused and fragmented, leaving services under-resourced and incapable of meeting needs. Reports (for example, Ritchie *et al.* 1994) emphasise paucity of provision and the impact of resource shortage on the appropriateness of discharge, placements, and follow-up support services.

The picture, though, is not entirely bleak. Barnes (1997) found that the Mental Illness Specific Grant had encouraged the development of innovative new services and the expansion of traditional provision. It had promoted partnerships between agencies, and prompted a growth in support to carers and an increased targeting of services on people with a severe mental illness. What is not specifically questioned, however, is the impact on service users of non-continuous provision, the grant appearing to stimulate short-term initiatives. Carpenter and Sbaraini (1997) concluded that service users involved in the Care Programme Approach felt included in their care and treatment and were better informed about services and their rights. Users felt that they had more choice, and there was a high level of agreement about care programmes. However, there were gaps in provision, especially evening and weekend services, and few service users knew about complaints procedures. It had proved difficult to move away from a diagnosis and service-led approach, and inter-professional collaboration remained weak.

A similarly mixed picture is reported elsewhere (for example Buckley *et al.* 1995; Wilson 1995; Newton *et al.* 1996). Although care management does appear effective in prioritising people with the most complex mental health needs, users and carers express varying opinions about assessment and services, and about information provision and coordination between agencies. Concerns remain about the availability of care plans to service users, carers and providers, and about the continuity and flexibility of care. Whatever the evidence of innovative practice, the statutory, policy and organisational context for practice with mentally disordered people may have become part of the problem.

Recreating mayhem?

Learning the Lessons (Sheppard 1996) makes depressing reading with its unerring focus on apparently regular deficiencies in mental health policy and practice. Its time frame – inquiry reports since 1969 – and the repetitive nature of their findings and recommendations, indicate a need to move beyond the question 'what?' and the grouping of results by professional or service user group setting, or by the focus of service provision, to the question 'why?'. Why are services experiencing such difficulties? Why are the lessons *still* having to be learned? Indeed, are there lessons underlying those reported still to be understood?

These are meta-questions: standing back to review the position, and to generate hypotheses which might introduce new information to facilitate systems change. One such hypothesis suggests that all tragedy is a failure of communication (Prins 1975). Systems tend to engage in more of the same, to repeat approaches to problems and solutions, even when they are clearly not achieving desired outcomes. To address this, meta-questions invite participants to reflect on processes of which they are a part, to look for the not-so-obvious. What, then, does such a line of enquiry suggest?

First order change

Inquiries into tragedies involving mentally disordered people focus on *text* – an individual situation – and seldom make the *context*, and the way it is experienced in practice, a subject for exploration and comment. Similarly, child abuse and major research inquiries have rarely acknowledged the social, psychological and economic factors which might impinge on practice, or debated the balance to be struck between autonomy and the use of coercion or protective powers, between needs and resources, and between rights and risks. The focus tends to be on the outputs of professional work, rather than the dilemmas which practitioners inevitably encounter in practice. Little account is taken of processes by which outputs are generated or the influence of other inputs, including the organisational context of professional work (Jones and Joss 1995). What then develops is a skewed notion of competence. Replacing an appreciation of the multi-faceted nature of competence is a reductionist, individualistic and fragmented model which obscures the influence of factors such as policies and procedures, decision-making systems, the nature of risk, organisational culture, inter-agency processes, and often contradictory societal values and expectations. Accordingly, complexity and ambiguity are lost, and the nature of practice remains essentially unchanged. The focus is on problem solving and concrete solutions, or first order change, to the neglect of complex interactions and relationship or second order change. Policy interventions are therefore likely ultimately to be ineffective.

Similarly, the revision of policy guidance, and the development of the statutory mandate and organisational structures, have focused on identifying the skills to be practised, or the regulations and procedures to be followed, or the implementation of service changes. They have not been accompanied by change in underlying relationships or power structures, or by a shift in perspective as a basis for re-focusing activity. One example is the promotion of partnership between service users and professionals. The concept of partnership in legislation and policy guidance is often narrowly defined. The user's voice may be stronger, but goals and services remain 'profession-dominated'. Power relationships have not been sufficiently reconfigured to achieve a different relationship between service users and workers (Braye and Preston-Shoot 1995).

Another example is the failure to move beyond repeated calls for more efficient communication between agencies at planning and operational levels to a fundamental review of the fragmented health and welfare system (DoH 1992; Faulkner 1994; Sheppard 1996; Robbins 1996; Leslie 1997). There is a bewildering number of agencies and professionals involved (SSI 1997) such that, while joint activity is increasing at operational and managerial levels, a strong joint approach to mental health planning and provision is difficult to achieve (Barnes 1997). As with child abuse (Reder *et al.* 1993), inquiries have not appreciated that communication is much more than the structured handling of information and its mechanical transfer from one agency to another. The fundamental obstacles originating in organisational structures and inter-professional relationships have not been addressed.

Consequently, the symptoms will reappear, as in repeated tragedies and incidents of abuse in residential care, because what drives the problem has been missed. The system has responded with more of the same – refined procedural guidelines and stronger exhortations for good practice – rather than looking at the nature of relationships involved, and the dilemmas, assumptions and structures surrounding practice.

Dehumanising individuals

Wardhaugh and Wilding (1993), reflecting on how social care can become corrupted through institutional and professional 'deformation', hypothesise that some groups come to be regarded as not fully human. The demonisation of young people or of mentally disordered people, or the categorisation of some welfare recipients as undeserving, are examples. Devalued by society, they are moved beyond the bounds of moral obligation. They are then vulnerable to gratuitous actions unrelated to any legitimate policy aim, or to the misguided pursuit of acceptable policy goals. This appears especially likely when staff too are dehumanised – accorded low status, or isolated and powerless organisationally. Echoing this, the Cleveland Report's statement (Butler-Sloss 1988) that 'the child is a person, not the object of concern' warns that systems can act as if people do not matter. Indeed, local authorities, in judicial review findings against them, have been criticised *inter alia* because their decision-making has lacked compassion and humanity (R v Staffordshire CC, ex parte Farley [1997]; R v LB Hammersmith and Fulham, ex parte M [1997]; R v Gloucestershire CC, ex parte Mahfood and Others [1997]).

The statutory mandate is implicated here. Government failure hitherto to implement either the Law Commission's proposals (1993; 1995) on protecting vulnerable adults, or the sections of the Disabled Persons Act 1986 concerned with user involvement and advocacy, convey the message 'you are not important'. The Mental Health (Patients in the Community) Act 1995 may contravene the European Convention on Human Rights and Fundamental Freedoms (Parkin 1996), since it erodes the rights of mentally disordered people to make decisions about where they live or how they occupy themselves. Christopher Clunis has been unsuccessful in his attempt to sue health and local authorities for breach of statutory duty (Clunis v Camden and Islington HA [1997]). It remains very difficult for service users to establish liability in negligence for an inappropriate standard of care (X and others (Minors) v Bedfordshire CC [1995]) when health and local authorities are deciding whether or not, and how to implement their statutory duties. Finally, community care and mental health law are constructed around powers and duties, principally given to social services departments, rather than rights for service users to, for example, informed risk-taking, procedural fairness, satisfaction of needs, and specific quality standards, or to dignity, choice and community presence, through which meaningful citizenship might be experienced (Braye and Preston-Shoot 1994). In light of this, it is perhaps not surprising that inquiries (Sheppard 1996) regularly report inadequate or un-acceptable service provision – a lack of facilities or alternatives, poor conditions in hospitals, a low priority accorded to mentally ill people, an inadequate range of accommodation or insufficient staff, inappropriate placements within and outwith hospital, and operational policies which fail to emphasise the primacy of acceptable professional practice, whatever the resource position.

Lack of resources is clearly a significant factor in this catalogue of failures and missed opportunities. Less tangible is the effect of resource constraint on staff, but demoralisation or disillusionment may follow from encountering needs which cannot be met or being unable to uphold the knowledge base and skills of a competent professional. Carpenter and Sbaraini (1997) found that workers were worried about the focus on lack of resources and the difficulty of implementing the Care Programme Approach in present budgetary constraints. Coupled with confusion about managers' expectations, pressures to conform, and cultures of fear (Mitchell 1996), practice can become characterised by suppression of criti-cism, routine, and an emphasis on difference from, rather than commonality with service users. This precludes a dialogue with service users who, correspondingly, do not feel engaged in a partnership. This may partly explain the detachment which allows questionable practice to become accepted, or agreed policies on good practice to remain unimplemented. It may also explain how organisations can become inward-looking, even dangerous, blocking out new ideas or a critical appraisal of how they are managing their mandate.

The Barclay Report (1982) argued that social workers were not robust enough in challenging the lack of control people have of their own lives, inappropriate forms of care, and structural or organisational injustices and inequalities. It did not analyse why, but explanations are not hard to find. Social work's predominant location in local authorities has meant the negotiation of multiple accountabilities. The challenge has been to hold the dynamic tension between delegated discretion and professional autonomy, and between politically determined employers' purposes, professional values, and the needs of service users. However, professional interests have become increasingly conflated with employer interests. One outcome has been that the balance or mediating role implied by multiple accountability has been undermined. Accountability to agency dominates over concern with social processes of exclusion and oppression, or advocacy for people who are vulnerable and on the margins (Adams 1990; Yelloly and Henkel 1995).

Autonomy, discretion and confidence have been further undermined by the imposition of national standards, division into purchasers and providers, and preoccupation with the management of resources. Eligibility criteria and procedures appear prioritised above relationships with services users (Onyett 1992; Grimwood and Popplestone 1993; Leslie 1997), such that social work is losing human contact as its core purpose (Drakeford 1996). The result can be the neutralisation of moral concerns, the depersonalisation of service users, and the undermining of moral responsibility, as practice reflects dominant organisational imperatives and political interests. Prescribed tasks and procedures are followed regardless of whether they are professionally, morally and/or legally suspect.

Inquiries are uncovering insufficient focus on therapeutic work with patients, irregular use of advocates, infrequent interviews in private, and an absence of culturally relevant services. Mental health service users and researchers also paint a picture of regimes dominated by purposeless daily activity and poor staff–patient relationships; characterised too by indifference to functional or managerial interactions, with a narrow approach to mental distress and a lack of attention to civil and human rights. There is unofficial coercion, limited understanding of oppression, a failure to consider the legality of proposed actions, and a failure to underpin relationships with autonomy and self-determination. Contact is often brief and cursory, the content of which is unsatisfactory, and there is neglect of personal narratives and experiences of inequality, together with stigma and labelling in mental health processes. Services are experienced as depersonalising and coercive (Braye and Preston-Shoot 1995; Rogers and Pilgrim 1995; Walton 1998). Interestingly – or depressingly – these trends are strikingly similar to the closed system found amongst nurses by Menzies (1970). As a defence against anxiety associated with the nature of the work, organisational structures become characterised by conformity to guidelines and by fragmentation of tasks. Individual anxiety has not been contained and the defences used to evade it become institutionalised in how tasks are then performed. Defensive practice, delusional certainty and directive authoritarianism (Preston-Shoot and Agass 1990) are examples of processes adopted to counteract insecurity.

The dehumanisation and depersonalisation of staff also emerge from inquiry reports (Ritchie *et al.* 1994; Sheppard 1996; Leslie 1997), with the following consequences:

- agencies failing to ensure proper supervision to enable professionals to reflect on practice;

- inadequate staff training, protection and support;
- inadequate staffing levels, leading to unbalanced workloads and insufficient time for reflection and liaison, and an inability to match case complexity to the experiences and skills of staff;
- inadequate policies and procedures as frameworks for guidance;
- little encouragement and constant change.

The outcome, for both service users and staff could be a vicious circle of internalised oppression. Powerlessness promotes negative self-evaluations, apathy and passive acceptance, which result in resigned acceptance and a belief in the futility of action, prompting negative evaluations by others and exclusion, so generating further experiences of powerlessness.

Images of mentally disordered people

Mentally disordered people can have a dislocating and distressing impact on practitioners, such that there is a reluctance or unease to work with them (Prins 1975). Practitioners can be subject to intense emotional pressures, which can dislodge them from a clear appraisal of patterns and processes in interpersonal and inter-agency work. If organisations do not contain anxiety and provide a holding environment where complex work dynamics can be scrutinised, a closed system may develop where practitioners will become slow to revise judgements and consider alternatives (Reder *et al.* 1993; Munro 1996). This reinforces the concern which should follow from findings about the inadequacy of staff support and supervision. If practitioners are unable to manage their own feelings about working with mentally disordered people, they will prove unable to help them face their feelings and experiences (Prins 1988). Equally, the situation will generate defence mechanisms which are aimed at evading anxiety but which become institutionalised in, for example, ritual task performance, distancing, detachment and denial of feelings, and inter-organisational conflict (Preston-Shoot and Agass 1990).

Perhaps these defence mechanisms underpin those images of mental health and illness which perpetuate a restricted view of mentally disordered people as less competent, high risk, more trouble and with limited potential to change or to work in partnership (Braye and Preston-Shoot 1995). There are, of course, individuals who are dangerous, who do need intrusive supervision (Prins 1988), and whose tendency to inflict injury on themselves and/or others is both unpredictable and untreatable. Nevertheless, any such judgement should be informed rather than based on stereotypes or umbrella categories (Forbes and Sashidharan 1997) – mentally disordered offender; mental health service user. Accordingly, practice must engage with how images of competence affect the process and content of the work.

However, mental disorder is often constructed around a negative stereotype of dangerous behaviour. While rooted in fear rather than fact (Braye and Preston-

Shoot 1997) – because few individuals are intrinsically dangerous (Prins 1975) – this is a powerful contributory factor to the extension of powers of control. It is a response which emphasises risk assessment, service coordination, and surveillance via supervision registers and supervised discharge, rather than questions the level and nature of service provision. Thus, there is a strong association between mental illness and violence in the media, even though the former is a poor predictor of the latter. The image perpetuated is of mad murderers at large because of a failing policy (Rose 1997), of individuals who require control. Structural inequalities and poverty receive less attention. Focus on the distortion of good practice, and the disabling of organisations, when decisions about provision are governed by resources rather than needs, has been displaced by an assumption that statute and regulation are what is needed.

Put another way, the danger may lie not in mentally disordered people so much as in the response to them. The unwanted feelings and anxieties which are generated by the behaviour of some mentally disordered people are not contained but are expelled, with condemnation of actions translating into hate towards the person and denial of personhood. The challenge becomes one of changing destructive attitudes and promoting positive concern and involvement with mentally disordered people. It lies in presenting complicated truths to counter simple falsehoods (Drakeford 1996).

Policy-making – chaos or coherence?

Simple falsehoods rather than complicated truths have characterised policy-making. Political and ideological considerations have driven policy, rather than a wider angle lens incorporating professional and service users' perspectives. This has had several outcomes. First, policy-making has undervalued the professional and service user knowledge base. Indeed, such has been the attack on professional thinking, and the links made therefrom, that professions like social work are 'under erasure' (Pietroni 1995) because of their potentially critical thrust. There is little dialogue about practice realities and dilemmas. Thus, for example, scepticism about the potential of supervised discharge orders, in the context of resource constraint and the inability of regulation to prevent tragedy, apparently went unheeded.

Second, concern with fundamental human issues of social justice, need and fulfilment has been overshadowed by a concentration on techniques and control. For example, the Criminal Evidence (Amendment) Act 1997 will allow non-intimate samples to be taken *without consent* from some detained patients. The Crime (Sentences) Act 1997 may limit the court's powers to send mentally disordered offenders to hospital, undermining the previous consensus on diversion from the criminal justice system, despite the potentially negative consequences that this will have. Similarly, key policy commitments such as empowerment, partnership, and needs-led assessments become devalued as principles for practice because the dilemmas of practice – needs versus resources, rights versus risks, protection versus autonomy – are encapsulated in, rather than solved by them. This is because they are presented as undifferentiated concepts, capable of multiple meanings. They conceal rather than illuminate the dilemmas with health and social care relationships, and obscure the different meanings and scope which various stakeholders will apply to them (Braye and Preston-Shoot 1992; Kaganas *et al*. 1995).

Third, policy-making is dominated by immediacy. It is result oriented rather than learning focused. Instead of policy harmonisation or cohesion, based on review and revision, policies proliferate, characterised by duplication of effort and conflict of initiatives. The Mental Health Act 1983 has not been reviewed subsequent to the reforms generated by the NHS and Community Care Act 1990. Community care law provides neither a continuing nor complete, coordinated or coherent framework. Confusion remains about the relationship between the Care Programme Approach, care management, and after-care (Section 117, Mental Health Act 1983). Less than one-third of local authorities have fully integrated the Care Programme Approach with care management (Barnes 1997) and it remains unclear how far integration extends through referral and allocation processes, and information and budgetary systems.

Imbalance

Policies are questionable if they neglect the complex worlds of service users and practitioners. One distinctive social work contribution here is its focus on 'the individual in situation', its ability to connect micro experiences with macro issues. It is a balance which has to be uniquely understood and struck in each situation. This balance is threatened.

People's mental health may deteriorate as much due to preventable social factors, for example, a failure to provide after-care services, as to disease processes. Awareness has increased of social factors in the aetiology and course of mental illness (Braye and Preston-Shoot 1995) but this is not reflected in policy-making or in the statutory mandate. What predominates is an assumption that people's needs arise because of genetic or biological factors, from identifiable biochemical processes which, once currently diagnosed, are treatable or containable, because of mental incapacity to make sound and safe decisions and to recognise risks and danger. These explanations are accompanied by negative stereotyping which contributes to and justifies the service response – intrusive supervision, assistance with adjustment, and a focus on functional ability and relationships.

Alternative social models widen the frame and promote an understanding of needs and experiences which move beyond individual pathology. The ability to participate fully, to regain control, and to live a 'normal' life is blocked by social structures. The focus then is on powerlessness and on an individual's social and economic position which impacts on and defines their experience. This context generates severe stress and may contribute to a vicious cycle of breakdown and drift. A comparison with child protection (Reder *et al.* 1993) sees abusive behaviour occurring at times of heightened tension in relationships between vulnerable people, against a background of chronic social and environmental stress.

Both models have contributions to make (Braye and Preston-Shoot 1995) but the gap between this understanding and the policy context is widening. Thus inquiries, when discussing good practice, occasionally refer to recognising *all* aspects of a patient's condition, rather than addressing only the immediate and obvious signs of illness. This is the exception, however. Similarly, the competence of key workers is framed around identifying and recording symptoms, maintaining contact, complying with legal duties, and recognising indicators of dangerousness. Focus on anti-discriminatory practice is largely restricted to the use of advocates, and specialists on 'race', and to the importance of culturally relevant services. The complex interaction of various forms of discrimination, with which mentally disordered people have to contend, is only infrequently addressed. Users frame, articulate and describe their problems in various ways (Rogers and Pilgrim 1995; Braye and Preston-Shoot 1995), reminding us that distress has many meanings over and above that implied by a psychiatric diagnosis. A substantial discrepancy often exists in the way professionals and users construe mental health problems.

Legalism

One major aspect of imbalance is the increasing reliance on legalism in policy. While law and guidance provide a framework for practice, both have been criticised by judges (R v Gloucestershire CC, ex parte RADAR [1995]), inquiries (Ritchie *et al.* 1994; Leslie 1997), and commentators (Prins 1996; Braye and Preston-Shoot 1997) for lack of clarity about tasks, standards and priorities. Nor do they address either the imbalance between escalating demands and decreasing resources, or the ambiguities of practice. Community care law remains confused on the degree to which needs, rights and resources control questions of service provision, and on the question of who is competent to make what decisions about people's lives, and by reference to what values (Braye and Preston-Shoot 1994). The very complexity of practice, for instance in balancing autonomy, empowerment and protection, suffused with dilemmas and choice points, assessment and analysis, means that when and how to intervene, and to what level, cannot be reduced solely to a rule book. Equally, law and guidance cannot guarantee risk-free practice. Arguably, registers and supervised discharge orders represent oversimplified responses to the complexity and dilemmas of practice and people's lives.

Similarly, procedures may hinder good workers by constraining flexible and sensitive practice and by pre-empting what is not on the list, without helping less effective practitioners. Blaug (1995) refers to procedurally led and standardised practice as a great failure which distorts face-to-face interaction which must be central to human caring. It is also likely to increase defensive practice (Prins 1996) and to inhibit the expression by practitioners of uncertainty, doubt and alternatives, thereby increasing the risk of dangerous practice. Legalism also assumes that the powers and duties expressed through statute and guidance are mirrored in agency procedures, when case law indicates that organisations often do not accurately interpret the legislative mandate or follow guidance (Preston-Shoot 1996).

Indeed, it is questionable whether the law is appropriate or sufficient to manage the complexities of health and social care practice. Supervision registers and supervised discharge orders alone will not protect people, reduce the level of concern, or improve the care people receive. Fundamental are the availability, quality and appropriateness of services. Moreover, the measures could prove counterproductive. Parkin (1996) questions how practitioners will ensure that supervised discharge orders end appropriately. He identifies the paradox that patients will be well enough for hospital discharge but not fit for discharge from supervision because this is necessary to prevent deterioration. He notes that it will be no easier to identify dangerous patients or those where statutory provision may be necessary to secure compliance. Two possibilities therefore emerge – overuse or underuse – with the implication that the orders will primarily benefit only those who are willing to cooperate anyway.

Conversely, as a basis for intervention the law requires evidence on a balance of probability and not, as Webb (1976) argued, on a list of 'maybe factors' dredged up on the basis of correlations which are not necessarily causally related. However, this potential corrective against abuse of power is constrained by the inadequate safeguards which legalism offers service users. The findings of complaints procedures are not binding, although any departure from them by an organisation must be warranted and reasonable (R v North Yorkshire CC, ex parte Hargreaves [1997]). Access to judicial review is discretionary. It focuses narrowly on decision-making and whether an organisation has approached its tasks legally, rationally and with procedural propriety. The Ombudsman may enquire more widely but the investigative process is lengthy, not guaranteed, and cannot require an organisation to amend its decisions. Finally, courts are reluctant to hold authorities accountable for breach of statutory duty. In contrast, there are no clear or enforceable standards of care, underpinned by legal rights to, for example, sufficient assistance within a reasonable time, the provision of written plans and regular reviews.

Another equally fundamental question is whether the law is empowering or oppressive. Whilst some legalism does promote practice aimed at counteracting discrimination, and at valuing difference, elsewhere the legal mandate can be seen as oppressive, either by commission or omission. It continues to marginalise 'the social' even though, as noted earlier, wider systems contribute to the difficulties that people experience. The personal and the political remain separated, with restricted scope to focus and comment on the whole areas of concern. More critically, naming as individual problems those which are rooted in wider systems, and recruiting professions to serve that end, is arguably unethical, and an abuse of power (Barry 1990; Jones 1993).

Equally, legalism can have iatrogenic consequences (Prins 1996) for both service users and professions, including:

- denying asylum to people because they appear 'untreatable' and yet a danger to themselves and/or other people;
- undermining the capacity of practitioners for individual thought and professional judgement (Pietroni 1995), and reducing the quality of decisions by weakening the sense of personal responsibility which professionals bring (Prins 1975);
- minimising the importance of professional skills, knowledge and understanding;
- appearing to substitute for well-informed, adequately resourced practice;
- undermining the importance, and confident exercise of autonomy and discretion;
- obscuring the fact that different courses of action can lead to similar outcomes;
- increasing the possibility of defiance, deception and lack of cooperation because of the use of coercion;
- making easier the allocation of blame and responsibility, thereby increasing defensiveness rather than promoting a learning culture (Reder *et al.* 1993; Parkin 1996);
- prejudicing inter-agency work by creating paranoia and protectionism about what agencies become involved in (Sandford 1995).

One problem with inquiries, as a reflection of how practice has increasingly become legalised and judicialised, is that enquiry becomes translated into apparently self-evident certainties. Yet any belief that understanding has been achieved rests, as Webb (1976) noted, on *post hoc* explanations with insufficient *a priori* reliability to be of use in any causal or predictive sense. Attention is directed away from how results are produced, understood and used, and from how a knowledge base and approach for practice are constructed. The imprecisions when assessing risk, and the difficulties in weighing the balance of probability or identifying premonitory behaviour and future dangerousness, struggle to counter the belief that risk is, or ought to be, a clearly identifiable phenomenon, predictable and preventable. How the balance should be struck between autonomy and the use of coercive or protective powers, between rights and risks, and between needs and resources, and the impact of that uncertainty on practitioners, appear less worthy of debate than the importance of detailed history taking, training, and the circulation of relevant information. Whilst these may reduce the likelihood of flawed intervention, they cannot guarantee good outcomes. Practice is seldom routine. Situations are complex and difficult to understand, rarely being amenable to prescribed or standardised responses. Outcomes are difficult to predict (Yelloly and Henkel 1995). It is important, therefore, to distinguish between avoidable and unavoidable mistakes (Munro 1996), or between the fault-lines in all human enterprises and the flaws relevant to services (Leslie 1997).

Muddled values

Surprisingly little attention is devoted in inquiries to what may be called 'values for practice', other than to reiterate the duty to disclose information (LASSL(94)4) when a real risk of danger to the public exists, and to promote the involvement of families and carers in meetings and information gathering. Values, as a foundation for ethical and effective practice, remain muddled, despite the fundamental dilemmas appearing over a century ago (Robbins 1996).

Confusion exists over the purpose of decisions – the balance between rights and risks, care and control. The Reed Report (Department of Health and Home Office 1992) recommended that mentally disordered offenders should receive quality care and proper attention to their needs, where possible in the community, with the minimum necessary security, and with the objective of maximising rehabilitation. These values appear at odds with the intentions embodied in the Mental Health (Patients in the Community) Act 1995, and the likely outcome of the Crime (Sentences) Act 1997. The former prioritises public confidence over patients' rights and, in extending social control of mentally ill people, appears to prefer order to freedom (Atkinson 1996).

Confusion exists also over who makes the decisions. As Prior (1992) notes, one contradiction is that highly trained approved social workers, but also nearest relatives, may make an application under the Mental Health Act 1983 for admission to psychiatric hospital of a person for assessment or treatment. Another centres on consent to treatment. The basic principle of common law is that any intervention requires real consent, based on adequate information and given without duress or undue influence. Capacity to consent derives from being capable of understanding what is involved. The quality of the decision is irrelevant to the capacity to make it. A person may be incompetent if they do not understand what is involved. An 'irrational' decision based on a value position must be distinguished from a decision based on wrong facts or delusions.

A mentally disordered person does not necessarily lack the competence to understand what is involved in a proposed treatment, say for physical ill-health (Re C [1993]). However, while the law accepts the possible counter-therapeutic effects of a decision competently taken about physical health, the converse is true about mental health. The Mental Health (Patients in the Community) Act 1995 implies that patients cannot make rational decisions about rehabilitation, treatment or occupation. Here the quality of their decisions, and not just their capacity to understand, has inevitably become relevant. A diagnosis of mental disorder disqualifies their competence to define their own interests, replacing it with a predictive professional opinion of harm and risk.

Similar difficulties arise with partnership and empowerment. In government guidance (DoH 1990; 1991), and within a traditional value base, empowerment has meant enabling and is an expression of individualism – the power to exercise choice and to purchase in a welfare economy regulated by market forces. Partnership is expressed through written agreements or care plans, consultation and involvement in decision-making, and accountability through complaints procedures. However, this serves to reinforce existing agency structures and professional power (Braye and Preston-Shoot 1995; Bland 1997) because decision-making is controlled by practitioners, and because the consequences for mental health service users of refusing to acknowledge professional authority far outweigh the reverse. Indeed, this consumerist approach arguably marginalises what users want by envisaging needs through a narrow perspective of available services.

A radical value base envisages empowerment and partnership as giving mental health service users greater control, power and autonomy. It moves beyond issues of service provision to questions of citizenship and people's status in society (Gomm 1993; Braye and Preston-Shoot 1995). While both approaches promote principles of dignity, choice and fulfilment, and seek to make professionals more responsive and accountable, their goals differ. The radical agenda is concerned with equality, the more traditional agenda with treating people better and with participatory practice based within officially sanctioned rules, procedures and structures. It does not explore the political context explicitly, nor does it consider how power has been used to define people's interests and choices.

Both traditional and radical approaches have contributions to make. At different times and for different people, an individual experience of distress and/ or the socio-economic realities of life will take centre stage. Equally, providing preventive and protective forms of care or treatment, where involvement, negotiation and choice are genuinely significant, and authority and reasons for decisions are openly discussed, can be empowering. However, the traditional value base will not achieve the goal (DoH 1991) of *all* service users enjoying the same rights of citizenship as other people, rights to self-determination and risk-taking with the minimum of restraint on that freedom of action. Services for mentally disordered people are additionally open to question ethically because often they reveal more about moral panics and social problem construction than about the needs of individuals, and because the concerns of the majority have been addressed in a manner which undermines the rights, and further oppresses, one minority group.

Values are central to preventing professional and organisational abuse of individuals. Best (1994) provides a list of ethics for decision-making on purchasing. These include understanding each person's full circumstances; promoting equity, justice and access to services; aiming for the best response to people's needs and wants; ensuring freedom from structural oppression and counteracting stigma; and recognising that everyone has a contribution to make in the community. A similar values statement exists for Approved Social Workers (CCETSW 1993). Problems arise because the principles conflate traditional and radical values without recognising the areas of difference, and are not always supported by the legal and policy mandate. Nor is there any consensus, for the values held by professionals may not be shared by service users and/or other social groups. What professionals may see as protective or in someone's best interests, may be experienced by others as oppressive or paternalistic (Braye and Preston-Shoot 1995). Equally, calls for practitioners to operate with suspicion and caution in some circumstances (Prins 1988) sit uncomfortably alongside such principles as respect for persons. Moreover, developments in public sector management, strongly influenced by policy reforms, have subordinated the moral authority of professionals to organisational and policy imperatives. Actions become correct if procedures and guidance have been followed. Finally, values can become problematic when they become fixed attitudes, closed to scrutiny. Asking questions, involving other professionals, or invoking statutory powers, have sometimes been avoided because of confusion about practising anti-oppressively or blanket adherence to a particular principle (Prins 1975; Davies *et al.* 1995). Arguably, then, 'failures' may indicate fundamental conflicts obscured by, yet underpinning, service provision.

Understanding and understandable practice

How might practitioners and managers respond to this context? Practice which is understanding and understandable requires a multi-professional forum which is confident in interacting with legislative and governmental systems, and active in initiating or contributing to debates about how welfare and justice are con-figured. There remain unresolved, challenging questions about the nature and purpose of health and welfare services, and their statutory foundations, for mentally disordered people. These cannot simply be explained away, or answered by inquiries or the use of undifferentiated concepts like partnership, choice or efficiency. When, how, how far, and for what purpose to intervene, remain at the centre of practice – questions of ethics, justice and rights, and how these should be realised. Social work has a justifiable political role here (Barclay Report 1982), whatever the attacks on its so-called 'correctness'. Thus, existing economic and social policies should not be taken as given, but assessed for their impact on people's lives. Professionals must be concerned with inequality, with the denial and menacing of civil liberties, and with unchecked government (Hutton 1997). Seedhouse (1988) refers to deliberation with integrity, weighing all relevant factors, and reflecting on the reasons for, and outcomes desired from action. Husband (1995) similarly refers to morally active practitioners who weigh up value choices and balance rights, risks and responsibilities, even when the result-ing intervention is at odds with prevailing orthodoxy. The aim is a moral intervention which prevents or eliminates obstacles to human potential, while also not causing harm to others. It differs fundamentally from the application of automatic rules or blanket policies. Healthy systems require ethically aware and active professionals who will adopt a sceptical position and engage in critical reflec-tion and analysis, who will challenge received ideas, ask awkward questions, and open up an exploration of possibilities. Organisations can empower employees by valuing practitioner and manager appraisal of roles, tasks and functions, and their relationship with wider socio-political questions.

One essential dialogue within and between health and social care organisations, and with policy-makers, centres on the competence of *organisations*. Key questions include:

- how to engage with the dilemmas posed by statutory mandates, time and resource shortage, and professional roles, and how to support practitioners to work in an empowering way;
- how agencies acknowledge the feelings which the work engenders and how they share responsibility with practitioners;
- how organisations, given that practice contains uncertainty, anxiety and ambiguity, can provide clear guidance about the principles which are to take precedence in practice, and resource practitioners through structures of support, supervision and training;
- how agencies can encourage practitioners to voice concerns, whether about the extent to which organisations adhere to values which should underpin health and social care, or about malpractice, or about organisational culture and established ways of working;
- how agencies can involve staff in establishing and reviewing goals, policies, and the objectives and procedures derived from them.

The focus here is both on providing a containing and holding environment, and accepting that accountability to an employer can only be fulfilled with integrity where it is consistent with the higher order principle of effective and ethical practice, defined by reference to core principles, and to the knowledge base which informs understanding.

A second dialogue concerns informed organisational and policy development. This involves reasserting policy leadership by:

- agenda building – articulating the moral, ethical and practice questions which a concern for people, their needs and rights generates, making practice and organisational issues visible;
- problem defining – articulating what is needed to do the job well;
- policy assessing – evaluating how policies benefit service users; analysing policies against criteria concerned with meeting needs, anti-oppressive practice, equal opportunities, and measurable outcomes;
- practice assessing – questioning whether practitioners and managers have a clear picture, what they might not want to see, what they believe to be happening and why;
- proposal making – including all stakeholders in developing services.

The skills required here are analysis – evaluating problems; politics – using power; interaction – working together; and clarification – of the values, knowledge and support required for well-informed practice. Practice here may include forming alliances with other organisations, and with service users, to advocate for change and to 'name the games' in social policy, particularly the implications for practice of funding decisions, imprecise legal mandates, and political stereotypes of welfare practice and service user groups.

It is into social, political, professional and organisational arenas that social work should take fundamental questions about the nature of the task, about services, and about responsibility. Thus, what risks can social workers take? What rights should people have, how should conflicting rights be balanced, and how might these rights be codified in statute? Given the inevitability of risk and uncertainty, when should professionals intervene? Decisions may appear reasonable on the evidence available (Munro 1996), so how should the tension between rights and risks, and care and control, be managed? What are acceptable standards of service provision, and are the risks acceptable which follow from workers and services being overloaded and under-resourced (Preston-Shoot and Agass 1990)?

A third dialogue concerns empowering and ethical practice. A key to empowering practice is to clarify what level of empowerment is being con-templated. Potentially disempowering aspects of intervention include the inability to influence decision-making, an unequal power balance, and a lack of control over what information is shared and the fear that information will be taken out of context. They also include the absence of information about procedures, disagreement with how facts are interpreted and insufficient time to discuss how problems are construed and solutions defined, and workers focusing on the content of work while users prioritise the degree of trust, support, caring and empathy within the process.

A further key to empowering practice must, therefore, be an acknowledgement of power and a determination to change power relationships. Practice should recognise the realities of how power is distributed in a relationship by:

- an open discussion of power, including rights of redress;
- a clear explanation of role – what is negotiable and non-negotiable, and why;
- clarifying who has what rights;
- providing information about the legal position;
- allowing space for the expression of feeling;
- identifying options and using written agreements to reflect decisions.

The objective is to develop a shared sense of purpose, and a relationship that does not oppress difference or abuse power differentials. This can be summarised in the following way:

Respecting individuality

- concern for people's value and rights;
- problem definition which addresses all aspects of a person's situation;

- identifying needs and wants, and setting quality standards for a person's care and development;
- offering space to negotiate about the purpose of involvement and the criteria by which success will be gauged;
- maximising choice areas;
- joint decision-making about what the issues are and how they will be tackled, to enable people to regain some control over their lives.

Counteracting imbalance

- thinking systemically, looking wider than the immediate and individual situation;
- recognising that changes and distress have multiple and complex causality;
- addressing structural issues which limit people's choices and which create or maintain isolation and exclusion.

Refocusing images

- challenging assumptions;
- avoiding the pitfalls of stereotyping or monoculturalism;
- examining interventions for their implications;
- using legislation to achieve change for service users.

Promoting second order change

- encouraging redefinition of issues;
- recognising that mental ill health is a powerful social construct;
- acknowledging people's strengths;
- encouraging collective action;
- sharing skills;
- connecting with other sources of power.

Empowering aspects of intervention include people feeling *able* to participate, through preparation and the use of advocates, the provision of accessible information and the opportunities to make real choices and to influence decisions, and through attention to the effects of oppression. Intervention should leave people feeling cared for as people, and should see them as subjects rather than objects – aiming to identify their stories, concerns and experiences, linking their personal expression of difficulties where appropriate with the wider context, and addressing issues of exclusion, isolation and disadvantage, all of which limit their choices. Although the concern should be to enable them, individually and collectively, to act as change agents by tackling internalised negative self-evaluations, developing support networks, and building on strengths, current practice retains some fundamental dilemmas or contradictions which practitioners and managers must attempt to reconcile. Prior (1992), for example, focuses on the organisational context and questions whether approved social workers can deliver less restrictive alternatives when they work in provider-led, cash constrained departments. She also queries how they can balance care and control, or act as advocates for mentally ill people while also having responsibility for public protection.

The challenge is to manage the 'solution space' (James 1994), and to reconcile or balance the competing interests and values within the mandate to practise. For example, the imperative of advocacy for mentally ill people, or the legislative requirement to provide the least restrictive alternative appropriate, must be met alongside recognition that the scope for advocacy may be limited by the social worker's employment location and the restricted choice of services available. In similar vein Darvill (1997) distinguishes between resolvable and unresolvable contradictions, and offers a six-point model of analysis and intervention. *Analysis* includes identifying personal bias in approaches to a dilemma or problem and reflecting on how this may need to be modified; ensuring that the problem is widely owned and evaluating what may be contributing to the dilemma, for example misinformation, lack of knowledge, problem retention mechanisms, or ambiguous terminology or behaviour. Analysis concludes with the consideration of alternative solutions. *Intervention* then consists of involving stakeholders in holding unresolvable contradictions, finding partial solutions where necessary, identifying unconscious as well as conscious behaviour, legitimating feelings of chaos and bewilderment, and providing support.

Some principles underpinning intervention have been articulated in law and guidance, namely access to information and to forms of redress, and procedural fairness – being involved in decision-making, and knowing the reasons for decisions. Anti-discriminatory practice also finds support in statute, to ensure that the law is not used disproportionately against already disadvantaged groups and to provide culturally relevant services. However, anti-oppressive practice, as challenging stereotypes and empowering people, remains, rather, a moral obligation.

At the same time some other principles will be *contested*. How to protect an individual's autonomy and self-determination in a context of someone deemed incapable of evaluating risk to themselves or others, or how to construe partnership in the context of compulsory admission to hospital, are examples. Like confidentiality or self-determination, they are open to qualification. However, to what degree, and for what reason they are qualified, requires careful articulation by reference to values and to a knowledge base. Similarly, some principles will generate *conflict*. That of social order, protecting the public from significant risk or harm, may conflict with principles of privacy, choice and community presence. Providing resources for one individual, to promote and maintain their physical and mental health, may conflict with principles of equity and proportionality. Others are difficult to judge, for instance prioritising those most at risk, or care and control in the context of the least restrictive alternative.

These instances demonstrate that models for managing the solution space are useful, so that practitioners and managers can reflect on the influence of personal and organisational values, can envisage the advantages and disadvantages of various options for action, and can articulate the values underpinning their judgements.

Conclusion

Welfare has frequently been presented as ineffective. This chapter's message, rather, is that the policy and practice context is problematic, and that the momentum created by incidents involving mentally disordered people has been used to minimise disturbance as much as, if not more than, to generate learning. The unpalatable fact is that the world is complex and unpredictable, that the best decisions do not necessarily result in the best outcomes, and that understanding is limited. Policy-makers and professionals, and those they represent, must contain anxiety, hold onto feelings of anger and fear, and build relationships through which learning can occur. Otherwise, the motives determining the future shape of policy and practice may be driven by an acting out of uncontained emotions, rather than by a calmer reflection on the human issues involved for staff and service users, the values which should underpin health and social care, and the core elements of good practice and a facilitating environment for that practice.

Cases

Clunis v Camden and Islington HA [1997] *The Times*, 10 December.
R v Gloucestershire CC, ex parte Mahfood and Others [1997] 1 CCLR 7.
R v Gloucestershire CC, ex parte RADAR [1995] CO/2764/95.
R v LB Hammersmith and Fulham, ex parte M [1997] 1 CCLR 69.
R v North Yorkshire CC, ex parte Hargreaves [1997] 1 CCLR 104.
R v Staffordshire CC, ex parte Farley [1997] 7 CL 186.
Re C [1993] NLJR 1642.
X and Others (Minors) v Bedfordshire CC [1995] 3 All ER 353.

Circulars

HSG(94)5: Introduction of Supervision Registers for Mentally Ill People.
LASSL(90)11: Caring for People – the Care Programme Approach for People with a Mental Illness Referred to Specialist Psychiatric Services.
LASSL(94)4: Guidance on the Discharge of Mentally Disordered People and their Continuing Care in the Community.
LASSL(95)12: Building Bridges.

References

Adams, R. (1990) *Self Help, Social Work and Empowerment*. London: Macmillan.
Atkinson, J. (1996) 'The community of strangers: supervision and the new right'. *Health and Social Care in the Community* 4 (2), 122–125.

Barclay Report (1982) *Social Workers, their Role and Tasks*. London: Bedford Square Press.

Barnes, D. (1997) *Monitoring the Use of the Mental Illness Specific Grant in 1994/95 and 1995/96*. London: Department of Health Social Services Inspectorate.

Barry, N. (1990) *Welfare*. Buckingham: Open University Press.

Best, D. (1994) *Purchasing and Contracting Skills*. London: CCETSW.

Bland, R. (1997) 'Keyworkers re-examined: good practice, quality of care and empowerment in residential care of older people'. *British Journal of Social Work* 27 (4), 585–603.

Blaug, R. (1995) 'Distortion of the face to face: communicative reason and social work practice'. *British Journal of Social Work* 25 (4), 423–439.

Braye, S. and Preston-Shoot, M. (1992) 'Honourable intentions: partnership and written agreements in welfare legislation'. *Journal of Social Welfare and Family Law* 6, 511–528.

—— (1994) 'Partners in community care? Rethinking the relationship between the law and social work practice'. *Journal of Social Welfare and Family Law* 2, 163–183.

—— (1995) *Empowering Practice in Social Care*. Buckingham: Open University Press.

—— (1997) *Practising Social Work Law*. 2nd edn. London: Macmillan.

Buckley, J., Preston-Shoot, M. and Smith, C. (1995) *Community Care Reforms: The Views of Users and Carers*. Manchester University of Manchester School of Social Work.

Butler-Sloss, E. (1988) *Report of the Inquiry into Child Abuse in Cleveland*. London: HMSO.

Carpenter, J. and Sbaraini, S. (1997) *Choice, Information and Dignity: Involving Users and Carers in Care Management in Mental Health*. Bristol: The Policy Press.

Casement, P. (1985) *On Learning from the Patient*. London: Tavistock.

CCETSW (1993) *Requirements and Guidance for the Training of Social Workers to be Considered for Approval in England and Wales under the Mental Health Act 1983*. London: Central Council for Education and Training in Social Work.

Cecchin, G. (1987) 'Hypothesising, circularity and neutrality revisited: an invitation to curiosity'. *Family Process* 26 (4), 405–413.

Commission on Social Justice (1994) *Social Justice: Strategies for National Renewal*. London: Vintage.

Darvill, G. (ed.) (1997) *Managing Contradiction and Avoidance*. London: National Institute for Social Work.

Davies, N., Lingham, R., Prior, C. and Sims, A. (1995) *Report of the Inquiry into the Circumstances Leading to the Death of Jonathan Newby (A Volunteer Worker)*. Oxford: Oxfordshire Health Authority.

Department of Health (1990) *Community Care in the Next Decade and Beyond: Policy Guidance*. London: HMSO.

—— (1991) *Care Management and Assessment: Summary of Practice Guidance*. London: HMSO.

Department of Health and Home Office (1992) *Review of Health and Social Services for Mentally Disordered Offenders and Others Requiring Similar Services*. (The 'Reed Report'). London: HMSO.

Drakeford, M. (1996) 'Education for culturally sensitive practice'. In S. Jackson and M. Preston-Shoot (eds) *Educating Social Workers in a Changing Policy Context*. London: Whiting and Birch.

Faulkner, A. (1994) 'Mission impossible'. *Community Care*, 8–14 September, 22–23.

Forbes, J. and Sashidharan, S. (1997) 'User involvement in services – incorporation or challenge?' *British Journal of Social Work* 27 (4), 481–498.

Gomm, R. (1993) 'Issues of power in health and welfare'. In J. Walmsley, J. Reynolds, P. Shakespeare and R. Woolfe (eds) *Health, Welfare and Practice: Reflecting on Roles and Relationships*. London: Sage/Open University.

Grimwood, C. and Popplestone, R. (1993) *Women, Management and Care*. London: Macmillan.

Husband, C. (1995) 'The morally active practitioner and the ethics of anti-racist social work'. In R. Hugman and D. Smith (eds) *Ethical Issues in Social Work*. London: Routledge.

Hutton, W. (1997) *The State to Come*. London: Vintage.

James, A. (1994) *Managing to Care*. London: Longman.

Jones, E. (1993) *Family Systems Therapy: Developments in the Milan-Systemic Therapies*. Chichester: John Wiley.

Jones, S. and Joss, R. (1995) 'Models of professionalism'. In M. Yelloly and M. Henkel (eds) *Learning and Teaching in Social Work: Towards Reflective Practice*. London: Jessica Kingsley Publishers.

Kaganas, F., King, M. and Piper, C. (eds) (1995) *Legislating for Harmony: Partnership under the Children Act 1989*. London: Jessica Kingsley Publishers.

Law Commission (1993) *Mentally Incapacitated and Other Vulnerable Adults: Public Law Protection*. Consultation Paper 130. London: HMSO.

—— (1995) *Mental Incapacity: Summary of Recommendations*. Consultation Paper 231. London: HMSO.

Leslie, A. (1997) *Practice, Planning and Partnership: The Lessons to be Learned from the Case of Susan Patricia Joughin*. Douglas: Isle of Man Government.

Menzies, I. (1970) *The Functioning of Social Systems as a Defence against Anxiety*. London: Tavistock.

Mitchell, D. (1996) 'Fear rules'. *Community Care* 14–20 March, 18–19.

Munro, E. (1996) 'Avoidable and unavoidable mistakes in child protection'. *British Journal of Social Work* 26 (6), 795–808.

Newton, J., Ryan, P., Carman, A., Clarke, K., Coombs, M., Walsh, K. and Muijen, M. (1996) *Care Management: Is it Working?* London: Sainsbury Centre for Mental Health.

Onyett, S. (1992) *Case Management in Mental Health*. London: Chapman and Hall.

Parkin, A. (1996) 'Caring for patients in the community'. *Modern Law Review* 59, 414–426.

Pietroni, M. (1995) 'The nature and aims of professional education for social workers: a post-modern perspective' In M. Yelloly and M. Henkel (eds) *Learning and Teaching in Social Work*. London: Jessica Kingsley Publishers.

Preston-Shoot, M. (1996) 'Contesting the contradictions: needs, resources and community care decisions'. *Journal of Social Welfare and Family Law* 18 (3), 307–325.

Preston-Shoot, M. and Agass, D. (1990) *Making Sense of Social Work: Psychodynamics, Systems and Practice*. London: Macmillan.

Prins, H. (1975) 'A danger to themselves and to others. Social workers and potentially dangerous clients'. *British Journal of Social Work* 5 (3), 297–309.

—— (1988) 'Dangerous clients: further observations on the limitation of mayhem'. *British Journal of Social Work* 18 (6), 593–609.

—— (1996) 'Can the law serve as a solution to social ills? The case of the Mental Health (Patients in the Community) Act, 1995'. *Med. Sci. Law* 36 (3), 217–220.

Prior, P. (1992) 'The Approved Social Worker – reflections on origins'. *British Journal of Social Work* 22 (2), 105–119.

Reder, P., Duncan, S. and Gray, M. (1993) *Beyond Blame: Child Abuse Tragedies Revisited*. London: Routledge.

Ritchie, J., Dick, D. and Lingham, R. (1994) *Report of the Inquiry into the Care and Treatment of Christopher Clunis*. London: HMSO.

Robbins, D. (1996) *Mentally Disordered Offenders: Improving Services*. (CI(96)20). London: SSI/DoH.

Rogers, A. and Pilgrim, D. (1995) 'Experiencing psychiatry; an example of emancipatory research'. In G. Wilson (ed.) *Community Care: Asking the Users*. London: Chapman and Hall.

Rose, D. (1997) 'Trial by television'. *Community Care* 4–10 December, 30–31.

Sandford, J. (1995) quoted in Rickford, F. 'Contrasting opinions'. *Community Care* (Inside Supplement), 30 November–6 December, 2–3.

Seedhouse, D. (1988) *Ethics: The Heart of Health Care*. Chichester: John Wiley.

Sheppard, D. (1996) *Learning the Lessons*. 2nd edn. London: The Zito Trust.

SSI (1992) *Implementing Caring for People: Assessment*. London: Department of Health.

—— (1997) *Services for Mentally Disordered Offenders in the Community: An Inspection Report*. (CI(97)19) London: Department of Health.

Walton, P. (1999) 'Psychiatric hospital treatment: a case of the more things change, the more they remain the same'. *Journal of Mental Health* (forthcoming).

Wardhaugh, J. and Wilding, P. (1993) 'Towards an explanation of the corruption of care'. *Critical Social Policy* 13 (1), 4–31.

Webb, D. (1976) 'Wise after the event: some comments on "A danger to themselves and others"', *British Journal of Social Work* 6 (1), 91–96.

Wilson, G. (ed.) (1995) *Community Care: Asking the Users*. London: Chapman and Hall.

Yelloly, M. and Henkel, M. (eds) (1995) *Learning and Teaching in Social Work*. London: Jessica Kingsley Publishers.

Zito, J. and Howlett, M. (1996) 'Introduction'. In D. Sheppard (ed.) *Learning the Lessons*. 2nd edn. London: The Zito Trust.

Chapter 6

Multi-agency risk management of mentally disordered sex offenders

A probation case study

Daniel Grant

Mental disorder and sex offending: some introductory considerations

The study of multi-agency case management in a context where the social control of dangerous and mentally disordered offenders is necessary reflects just one of Herschel Prins's contributions to a literature which studies the complex inter-actions between mental disorder and criminality (see for example, Prins 1986, 1995).

This chapter examines multi-agency case management, first by identifying the benefits it offers and second, by examining the case history of a mentally disordered sex offender who became a subject in an experimental case management project. In conclusion, the advantages of a coordinated response to the risk that dangerous and mentally disordered sex offenders present to the public are discussed.

Mental disorder and sex offending, albeit that both may cause public and professional concern, are distinct aspects of human experience and behaviour, each demanding specialist intervention. Many popular perceptions of both are based on confusion and ignorance, generated from myth and stereotype, sustained by contemporary images of twentieth-century folk devils (see for example Richardson *et al.* 1991; Goode and Ben-Yehuda 1994), and reinforced in exaggerated form by media accounts and popular entertainment. Moral panics, often ignited by a single and unusual case, can sway public opinion away from the desire to understand towards punitive solutions based on social exclusion, with deviance amplification a likely consequence (among numerous classic texts of the sociology of deviance see in particular Lemert 1967; Mankoff 1971; Young 1971; Cohen 1985). But while it may be more comfortable for public and politicians alike to dissociate themselves from behaviour which causes such revulsion than to regard it as a problem requiring treatment or management, it is also the case that newspaper profits associated with this revulsion are funded by that same public, with a seemingly insatiable appetite for both lurid description and prurient condemnation. Hence the monsters, beasts, loonies and perverts of the tabloid press become the patients or clients of the professionals, and the subjects of books such as this one.

Not all mentally disordered people commit sexual offences, nor do sex offenders as a group manifest higher rates of psychiatric illness, personality disorder or learning disability than the population in general (see, for example, Barker and Morgan 1993; Fisher 1994). Because the association between mental disorder and sex offending, therefore, which is neither clear to grasp nor simple to manage, occurs at the point of overlap between distinct areas of concern, informed and sensitive negotiation of competing issues and priorities is required of the professionals concerned. For example, risk, civil liberties, public protection and treatment all demand attention, not only because each has the potential to extinguish or ignite the dangerousness of the offender (an empirical point), but also because each carries within it a piece of social or political philosophy about the proper management of people whose behaviour and way of being defy comprehension. Such philosophical disagreements transcend empirical evaluation, and almost no position can therefore simply be dismissed as 'wrong'. As Herschel Prins has steadfastly maintained, when sex offending and mental disorder converge, because no single discipline is capable of dealing with – or even grasping – all the issues which arise, the need for coordinated multi-disciplinary case management is accordingly paramount.

For this and other reasons, professionals dealing with mentally disordered sex offenders must rely on experience as well as legislation, policy and research to determine if a person's behaviour (and the level of risk it poses) are more appropriately addressed by mental health, criminal justice, or some combination of the two. Despite legal and psychiatric developments the question 'mad or bad?' can never produce an answer applicable to all individual cases, but rather one which offers a framework definition to guide local policy and professional judgement in relation to specific cases. It is in good part for their appreciation of this point and their facilitation of discussion about how to formulate this policy and judgement, that Herschel Prins's contributions have been so influential among professionals at all levels of seniority.

The purpose and character of multi-agency intervention with mentally disordered sex offenders

It follows from these considerations that when dealing with mentally disordered sex offenders on a multi-agency basis, it is essential to understand and agree the priority purpose of professional involvement, given that each agency has separate tasks and responsibilities, emphases and cultures, procedures and preferences, funding and accountability. These differences unavoidably underpin the common purpose of controlling problematic behaviour through treatment, management, incapacitation or some combination of the three, and, unless acknowledged and dealt with on a day-to-day basis, can lead to differences in practice, or even conflict.

This chapter's concern is not with treating mental illness but with the control of that form of illegal behaviour defined as sex offending. A range of controls is available to professionals, from therapeutic services based on moral persuasion (such as the cognitive behavioural programmes currently so popular with the probation service and other protective agencies) right through to, at the other extreme, forms of imprisonment or secure provision which sever, at least temporarily, contact between offender and public. The former might, a little crudely, be categorised as trading the present security of incapacitation for the hope of future change; the latter, while normally entailing therapy as well as incapacitation, faces three main problems.

First is the therapeutic problem that faces all institutional therapy that, geographically and experientially, it occurs at a distance from the location of the crimes; second, there is the practical problem that, therapy being a secondary consideration to incapacitation, there is little chance to test its efficacy until the offender is discharged; and third, particularly where the incapacitation is within the criminal justice system, it is seldom possible to link the discharge date to response to therapy, because the former is determined by predominantly non-therapeutic considerations. A similar problem applies more generally to attempts to introduce a therapeutically driven reward system into a penal institution propelled by its own rules, culture, logic and routine.

This being so, and given a reasonably widespread belief that prison, for all its punitive and prophylactic utility, is either neutral or damaging to criminals' character or behaviour, in cases other than the most extreme, there is always likely to be judicial interest in community control; and even where prison is chosen, such control may well follow it, especially given the increasing confidence that something at least 'works' in supervision (McGuire 1995).

Multi-agency supervision has developed both from the recognition that working together can enhance task performance, and the political necessity of criminal justice and other public service agencies being seen to demonstrate improved effectiveness. Work based on collaboration and shared responsibility is increasingly seen as the most effective method of supervising mentally disordered sex offenders in particular, and in recognition of the complex and multi-disciplinary issues (across the boundaries of health, medicine, social service, education, police and probation) which arise in this field, collaborative structures increasingly exist to coordinate activities and advise on local policy. This means that when, as they inevitably sometimes do, things go wrong, lessons can be both learned and communicated, and responsibility comfortingly shared.

Further, the priority given by statute and professional culture to protection from sex offenders is sufficiently powerful and widespread to override many of the differences of emphasis – between, for example, civil liberty and public protection, or confidentiality and communication – that militate against inter-agency collaboration in other spheres of activity such as personal drug use or minor benefit fraud. So in the case of mentally disturbed sex offenders, the shared aim of protection from sexual violence serves as a powerful unifying symbol for mental health and criminal justice agencies, overriding many of the cultural and statutory differences between them. It necessitates and facilitates the sharing of intelligence and effort in a manner so designed to meet an agreed aim as to enable lesser differences in agency, method and philosophy to be put on ice.

Multi-agency case management has focused, for probation in particular, on a concern with risk (see Kemshall 1996), and is referred to here as multi-agency risk management. Since so far no agency has emerged to offer to coordinate this activity – or if it has, it has not achieved legitimation from the other players – and because legislative responsibilities are less clearly spelt out than they are in the case of, say, child protection, there is widespread local variation in the respective activities of partner agencies, and often relative weakness in planning, monitoring and evaluation.

It could be argued that the probation service, being involved in managing mentally disordered sex offenders through community supervision, would be well placed to assume such a role; and so to a degree it would. After all, the statutory purpose of supervision under a probation order is defined in Section 2(1) of the Powers of Criminal Courts Act 1973 (as substituted by Section 8(1) of the 1991 Act) as securing the rehabilitation of the offender, protecting the public from harm from the offender, or preventing the offender from committing further offences (Home Office 1992a); and, against this background, strategies for probation work with sex offenders have been developed and two main aims identified – the protection of the public through effective supervision and the reduction of the risk of re-offending (Home Office 1992b).

None the less, these strategies do little to operationalise probation work; indeed, their breadth offers such scope for individual interpretation and variation of emphasis that anything from providing a social work service to concentrating on community protection initiatives can be justified. Given this wide availability of valid intervention strategies and the relative privacy of worker–offender inter- actions (Pithouse 1987), a certain 'artful consonance' is available to the probation service, in which the mandate to protect the public by rehabilitating the offender can be advanced simultaneously. This suggests that if the proper role of probation in any multi-agency initiative is to be developed, it is entirely appropriate to return to the service's core traditional function, namely rehabilitation.

Rehabilitation and treatment revisited

Rehabilitation is clearly a legitimate concern of the probation service, and has once again come to the forefront in discussions about the effectiveness of the probation service in view of recent interest in investing both financially and professionally in the 'what works' approach to practice (McGuire and Priestley 1995; Roberts 1995), after a decade in which it was overshadowed by diversion (see Raynor 1996; Mair 1996) or punishment.

Rehabilitation refers to much more than delivery of social work help to offenders: 'rehabilitation is a change in the offender's attitude, produced by the state intervention due to his criminal conviction and resulting in a willingness to

refrain from criminal acts' (Clear and O'Leary 1983: 18). To Clear and
intervention may derive from a number of factors which motivate the o
refrain from further crime, including the fear of being caught and punish
receiving insight into any emotional causes of criminal behaviour, and ̲g̲a̲i̲n̲i̲n̲g̲
access to socially legitimate opportunities. In short, the desired aim of
rehabilitation is that the offender chooses to refrain from committing further
offences.

Rehabilitation is not, however, a universally fashionable concept. May and
Vass (1996) for example, claim that it is now a thing of the past; but their model
of 'rehabilitation' is based largely on a model of individual casework designed to
correct the psychological maladjustment once thought to be the primary cause of
offending behaviour. This, however, ignores the extent to which rehabilitation is
increasingly sought by means such as social skills training, and reminds us, as if
we needed reminding, of the importance of clearly defining opaque concepts such
as 'rehabilitation': meanings change over time and place, and are by no means
impervious to political considerations.

For example, McWilliams (1986) documents the emergence of control in
the professional arena, as political, economic and social pressures have caused
successive governments to question and modify methods used to deal with
crime and criminal behaviour. From the early 1980s onwards, new cost-effective
methods of crime control were sought, and control, whether custodial or not, has
become a favoured response to all crime, not least of the sexual kind.

Control, however, is seen by some (Lacey *et al.* 1983; May 1991; Vass 1982)
as undermining the professional therapeutic approach to offenders, replacing
it with what is described as a punishment–administrative approach; and by
others (Harris 1992) as raising tensions for the probation service involving care
and control, liberation and constraint. But in truth the distinction between care
and control is less clear or precise than these writers imply. As well as creating
access to socially legitimate avenues of success, for example through learning
social skills and acquiring a heightened emotional awareness and self-control,
motivation to refrain depends on factors such as fear of detection and restriction
of opportunity, and there is no reason why acknowledgement of this within
probation supervision, and accordingly the adoption of these elements of crime
control, should present professional or ethical difficulties. Indeed, as we shall see
from the case example discussed later, probation supervision can harness many
forms of control to effect productive community supervision and multi-agency
case management of mentally disordered sex offenders.

The first step is to acknowledge that working with sex offenders is ultimately
about rehabilitation, but rehabilitation as broadly defined by Clear and O'Leary
above. If reduction in recidivism can be achieved by persuading the offender to
refrain from creating further victims, then so much the better. If there are doubts
about the offender's motivation to refrain from offending, and healthy scepticism
is the bread and butter of those who work in criminal justice, further help can
be provided for the offender through reducing opportunities for offending and

raising awareness of the possibility of detection. To increase motivation to refrain from offending is a necessary aim for the probation service, and this remains, in essence, rehabilitative. As Young has noted, however:

> Traditionally . . . a therapeutic approach to policy has contrasted with an emphasis on deterrence . . . Such an opposition has no logical basis, for if positivism is based on a motivational structure generated by punishments and rewards in the process of primary socialization, there is no reason why such punishments and rewards (including deterrence) should not be effective in later life.
>
> (Young 1994: 98)

Other professional agencies share the same aims as probation. Appreciating this and having the will to work with other agencies to prevent offending are the foundations of multi-agency crime prevention. Probation, with its responsibility for statutory supervision and redress to the courts in the event of non-compliance is, however, pivotal. The service acquires on a daily basis a wealth of intelligence about sex offenders, the value of which to other agencies is not to be under-estimated; but the same applies in reverse, for the potential contribution of agencies such as police, mental health and social services to probation supervision is immense. This is scarcely surprising, since they are all doing different parts of the same job, and only together can they complete the jigsaw.

Completing the jigsaw entails sharing not only intelligence and operational tactics (crucial as this is), but clinical knowledge, and being willing to revise methods in the light of external advice. Such advice may improve effectiveness and reduce the likelihood of public money being wasted on futile activity. For example, during July and August 1995, probation officers supervised 7,109 sex offenders (Association of Chief Officers of Probation 1996), an average of 132 per service, of whom 3,080 were on post-release supervision or community sentences. However, the service had the capacity to provide treatment pro-grammes for less than 65 per cent of these offenders, a situation in which the need for precise targeting is self-evident; but less than half these programmes involved relapse prevention instruction, and those which did not were considered by the Government's STEP Research Team (Beckett *et al.* 1994) to be unlikely to be effective with serious sex offenders. Hence, while the supply of community supervision was insufficient to meet demand, a large majority of convicted sex offenders on supervision in 1995 were receiving at best dubiously effective and at worst no treatment. One can only wonder whether a closer involvement between probation and the psychological or psychiatric services would have improved the former's rehabilitative performance and hence increased public safety. No agency has a monopoly on expertise, and probation officers are not infrequently invited to operate forms of clinical therapy in respect of which their training is less than comprehensive.

Enhanced supervision

While rehabilitation is the ultimate aim of managing mentally disordered sex offenders, and while acknowledging that the word 'treatment' covers (and so collapses) multitudinous forms of variably effective 'talking cures', it would be wrong to assume that rehabilitation is normally achieved by treatment. First, treatment of any kind is not reliably effective in the case of all (or even most) sex offenders, and any public confidence it enjoys is based on unrealistic expectations of its reductionist potential. Second, willing cooperation is required from the offender for statutory therapeutic intervention to have any chance of success; and while, given the circumstances in which it is normally sought, such cooperation is unlikely to be withheld, the scope for subtle non-compliance is self-evidently considerable. It is, after all, an enduring irony (if not contradiction) of treatment that much of its success depends on the honesty of the dishonest, and in particular on the dishonest becoming honest prior to and as a precondition of treatment, not as a consequence of it. Third, as treatment to a large extent takes place in a treatment room, relapse prevention, a crucial component of relatively successful programmes, must be discussed in the abstract, and is too seldom informed by the more complete, accurate and better informed portrayal of risk provided by agencies working in the offender's own community.

Enhanced supervision, on the other hand, refers to the use of external controls to reduce the likelihood of an offence being committed by an identified offender, and has been shown to produce impressive results (Grant 1998). At its simplest, since it does not entail any additional requirement for psychiatric treatment or alcohol and drug treatment it may be applied without consent to any offender through the existing statutory supervisory framework; but it can also, with consent, be extended beyond the offender's statutory involvement with probation. Enhanced supervision involves a partnership of (potentially) education, health, social service and criminal justice agencies, based on their willingness to transcend their own responsibilities by focusing collectively on the shared objective of public protection. Whereas in treatment the key figure is the offender, on whose trustworthiness and therapeutic malleability much depends, the important figures in enhanced supervision are the professional employees of these agencies; and the key to success is trust and communication between them in order to provide a more reliable source of information on which to manage the level of risk presented by the offender. The offender and his activities remain the central focus, but no gambles are taken on, or assumptions made about, an offender's trustworthiness; indeed, the offender ceases to be the *subject* of treatment, becoming instead the *object* of enhanced supervision.

It would not, however, be correct to see enhanced supervision and treatment as separate initiatives deriving from opposite ends of probation officers' continuum of intervention strategies. There is no theoretical or practical reason why, in suitable cases, the latter should not form a part of the former, and every reason for it to do so if this is helpful in a particular case. In managing the crimes of mentally disordered sex offenders, however, treatment, while doubtless sometimes necessary, is seldom sufficient.

Sex Offender Risk Management Approach (SORMA)

The potential of the enhanced supervision of mentally disordered sex offenders requires closer analysis and evaluation, however, and the following case example demonstrates a working model of how the probation service can facilitate and coordinate a multi-agency community supervision programme for sex offenders. What is more, as the offender concerned is mentally disordered, we shall see how the agencies involved worked together to protect the public. This case is one of six studied in considerable detail in 1995 during the experimental Sex Offender Risk Management Approach (SORMA) project (see Grant 1998).

SORMA lies at the core of this exploratory research project into the community supervision of men convicted of sexual offences. It is a system of multi-agency risk management of sexual offenders in the community, which aims to utilise the most convincing contemporary approaches to the control and treatment of sex offenders. SORMA is not, however, a simple re-arrangement of these existing components, nor does it simply add to the prevailing, and, some might say complacent, quasi-therapeutic treatment orthodoxy; rather, it disturbs it to offer reconsideration of the aim and purpose of the work, finding a broader context in which to examine these existing interventions.

SORMA has seven key components, and examples of how these transcend current practice emerge in the case study detailed below:

1   It is *unambiguously concerned with social control.*
2   None the less, it also entails *clinical treatment and therapy.*
3   It is centrally an aspect of *situational crime prevention.*
4   It involves *actuarial risk assessment and management.*
5   A key component is *surveillance.*
6   Crucial to its success is *multi-agency collaboration.*
7   Necessary to its success is the *maximisation of legislative authority.*

SORMA is concerned not with aetiology but with management, and in this sense is located within what Young has called the emerging tradition of new administrative criminology (Young 1994). The model, however, is also situated in and draws part of its value from an interaction between therapeutic ambition and environmental manipulation, though since the model also entails the repudiation of the distinction between supervision and therapy, its main focus is more on management and creating conformity than on humanistic self-expression: after all, in therapeutic sessions with controlling but 'caring' professionals, subjects can reveal much that they would conceal in the course of police interrogation. Extending the circle of confidentiality in this way appropriately transforms therapy into an instrument of public protection and control over those who would otherwise seek to impose their own oppressive forms of power over those more vulnerable than themselves.

Case study: Peter

Peter was 29 years old and lived in a housing association hostel with minimum support. He was subject to a 2-year probation order for the indecent assault of two teenage girls in separate incidents, with a condition to submit to psychiatric treatment, reside where directed, and attend the sex offenders' group run by the probation service.

Peter had a history of mental ill-health. He suffered his first mental breakdown at the age of 21 years and was admitted to an acute psychiatric ward, where he remained for 4 weeks. At this time he was having visual and auditory hallucinations, which mainly involved the devil plotting against him and God. He was made the subject of a Mental Health Act section order and diagnosed as suffering from schizo-affective psychosis. He was admitted on three subsequent occasions, for a maximum of 3 months, for the same problem. He had never been involved in a long-term relationship and had no dependent children, describing himself as a 'virgin' and blaming mental ill-health for denying him the confidence to start a relationship. He had experienced short periods of employment, but none for the last six years due to ill-health. At school he had been quite bright, and his psychiatrist described his cognitions as 'intact'. Indeed, when discussing his family background, Peter was able to remember the full names of 64 extended family members and the dates of birth of 31 of them (of whom 26 were children). He disclosed no evidence of being the victim of sexual abuse.

Peter had no previous convictions of any kind, though he had received a police caution in 1992 for indecently assaulting his 7-year-old nephew, an incident in which he undressed the boy and rubbed his erect penis against the boy's buttocks before, bizarrely, rolling the boy up in a carpet, for reasons which remained unclear.

The current offences began when he accosted two teenage girls who were walking along a street together. He stood very close to one of them and began to sing a love song to her. He then began to make sexually suggestive remarks to her, shouted obscenities and stroked her face and breast, over her clothes, with his hand. She was able to walk past him to summon help, and while she did so, he continued to shout obscenities.

The second incident occurred on a bus, three months later. He was on the top deck of the bus with several other passengers situated around him. He noticed two teenage girls (14 and 16 years) sitting together talking. He stared at them for a while and then moved to take up the seat directly in front of them. He leaned over the seat and started to make suggestive remarks. After inviting both girls to become his sexual partners, he focused his attention on the younger girl, and started to tell her how he would like her to come back to his room and have sex with him. He became aggressive while saying this and had placed his face very close to the girl's face. He was shouting at her and then pushed her backwards against the seat.

On both occasions, the victims had been in a public place and it had been daylight. There is no evidence to suggest that Peter had planned the encounters, beyond opportunistically drawing himself closer, once he had seen them. Members of the public had witnessed the offences, but none had intervened. Both incidents were immediately reported to the police, and Peter was arrested for both offences, after being identified from descriptions given by victims and witnesses. He readily admitted the offences, describing both as attempts to 'chat up' the girls that had gone terribly wrong. It is probable that he had contemplated accosting girls in similar public situations to those where the offences occurred, and indeed that he had previously done so: he was known to have been behaving in an aggressive way, at least periodically, for a considerable time, and to have been verbally abusive to vulnerable people. His targets were usually elderly people, young women or girls, and his preferred locations anywhere which the vulnerable might frequent.

Once he had selected his target, his behaviour was broadly predictable. In the case of a sexually motivated accosting, he would make a confrontational approach and use inappropriate language and actions to try and impress. When realising, soon after commencement of his actions, from the fact that the victim was uncomfortable and affronted, that his advances were unwelcome, he would, in a curious form of courtship disorder (Freund 1990), interpret this as a form of sexual or aggressive provocation and become aroused.

Such a theory fails to explain his motivation for abusing his nephew, however, an incident which added a pederastic dimension to his offending. During assessment for the sex offender group Peter revealed a strong sexual attraction to children, particularly boys, and though, following his caution, he seems to have contained his behaviour towards children, he presented as a paedophile with a preference for boys. When interviewed by the police for his offences against the girls, one of the first things he said was: 'I've been talking to my community psychiatric nurse about my illness, having to cope with stress and frustration as well as wanting to actually get somebody myself, make a relationship myself.' It is possible that Peter was doing just that, and that his anger was fuelled by his sense of failure, clumsiness and lack of genuine sexual motivation towards his victim.

The probation officer writing the pre-sentence report for the magistrates' court warned that all professionals involved with Peter were concerned that his offending could escalate in seriousness. Indeed, Peter, who showed clear signs of confusing attraction/lust with anger/intimidation, had expressed this concern himself, revealing fantasies of rape and claiming that he targeted his current victims because they resembled the girls in these fantasies. It was certainly reasonable to assume that, driven by these same fantasies, he might carry out more serious offences, and the author of the report assessed the risk of his re-offending as very high. A psychiatric report, obtained at the request of the defence solicitor, did not inform the court of any issues relating to risk.

In February 1995, as part of Peter's supervision and involvement in SORMA, a multi-agency risk management meeting was convened. This was attended by a psychiatrist, community psychiatric nurse, detective constable, principal social worker, hostel manager, hostel key worker, two co-working probation officers and Peter, who joined the meeting shortly after it had started. The meeting began with the psychiatrist outlining Peter's case history. The psychiatric services did not provide specific treatment, therapy or supervision for sexually abusive behaviour, but medication had been prescribed for his psychiatric illness. The community psychiatric nurse monitored Peter's behaviour and had offered counselling in times of crisis. The psychiatrist was asked if libido-suppressant drugs had been considered for Peter, and after discussion, it was decided this would be pursued with Peter. The principal social work practitioner was anxious to learn of any contact Peter might be having with children, and the police were concerned with preventing and detecting any crime related to his behaviour. This preliminary discussion helped to establish a range of concerns relating to Peter's behaviour, and set the agenda for the rest of the meeting.

Peter then joined the meeting and acknowledged the concern expressed about him, agreeing that the risk of his committing another similar offence was high. At this point, the psychiatrist introduced the idea of prescribing a libido-suppressant drug as a form of treatment, which might, along with the sex offender treatment programme and professional surveillance, reduce the likelihood of his re-offending. Peter expressed a willingness for such treatment, and the psychiatrist agreed to arrange an appointment for him to discuss this further. The meeting lasted for approximately one hour, with Peter present for half that time. The meeting had discussed inviting a relative of Peter's to become involved in super-vision (the involvement of relatives, friends or neighbours in the control network being a potentially vital aspect of SORMA), but no suitable person was identified.

It was important to establish a shared understanding of how his psychiatric condition and offending were linked. It was agreed that the best approach would be to regard Peter as an offender with the capacity to rape women and children. Indeed, he recognised this himself, and described rape fantasies. It appeared that aggression raised his sense of arousal, as did fear and intimidation in his victim, and that the schizo-affective psychosis aggravated this, so increasing the risk of violent attack. The mental disorder was controlled to a degree by medication but was considered unlikely to be cured or to remit. A starting point for the case management had been formulated with a universally understood and agreed joint assessment of which Peter was aware and to which he had contributed. The challenge was to test SORMA's suitability for an offender requiring considerable health and social service intervention. Would the statutory supervisory function provide too great a challenge for the care and welfare philosophy that often dominates these agencies, so detracting from the concern with risk, surveillance and crime prevention?

A risk management plan was negotiated, which included the following provisions:

- Peter would be actively discouraged from accosting vulnerable people to the extent that when it was discovered, the police would deal with the matter accordingly. All such matters were therefore to be reported to the police immediately they came to light.
- The probation officer would apply to the magistrates' court for a variation to Peter's probation order, restricting his contact with children. The wording of this variation would be agreed after seeking legal advice.
- Peter would be supported in his use of Cyproterone Acetate as a libido-suppressant drug.
- The key worker from the hostel would be regarded as Peter's most significant member of the community, as that person had most contact with him.

In March, Peter was served an eviction notice from the hostel. The staff consulted the probation officer about this, but were clear about their reasons: his behaviour had deteriorated generally, and while no specific trigger incidents had occurred, he had continued to seek out a female member of staff, a middle-aged woman, and harass her. The staff believed he presented a danger to her and determined that he would have to leave.

At this point, a number of problems were encountered. First, while the psychiatrist was able to start Peter on libido-suppressant medication almost immediately, the drugs had to be discontinued when a liver function test revealed an adverse reaction. Second, in April a decision was made not to pursue the variation of his probation order, as he was not able to demonstrate a clear enough understanding of the condition for his consent to be valid. And third, in May the hostel staff decided to enforce his eviction notice at the end of the month, giving Peter only three weeks to find another address. Numerous attempts had been made to try and find suitable accommodation, but to no avail; a community care assessment which had been completed failed to take into account his accommodation needs.

Peter was evicted from the hostel in early June and quickly found himself a bedsit. He introduced the owner to the probation officer, so that they could discuss his risk of offending. The probation officer viewed the property, which seemed suitable. The full range of concerns was divulged to the owner, with Peter's agreement. Links between her and the professionals involved were encouraged, and each professional was notified of Peter's change of circumstances in writing.

Within four weeks of moving into the bedsit, the owner contacted the probation officer: Peter had accosted a young girl on a bus and the child had to be escorted home. He had also knocked an elderly woman over by walking into her, and while it was not clear if this was deliberate, he had become verbally abusive to the woman and onlookers. The police had not been called, and the incident was only reported to the probation officer because of the surveillance of the landlady.

These incidents realised some of the concerns expressed at the risk management meeting. After detailed discussions between the probation officer and the principal social worker, police and community psychiatric nurse, it was decided that Peter should be seen by the new consultant psychiatrist (her predecessor having changed jobs). Peter went to the accident and emergency unit of the local hospital, and the duty psychiatrist was called. Given the nature of the risk outlined in the risk management plan handed to the psychiatrist when she arrived, he was admitted to the psychiatric unit for assessment, initially as a voluntary patient. Following a psychiatric case conference attended by the majority of those concerned with his case management, he was made subject to Section 3 of the Mental Health Act 1983, and a forensic psychiatric assessment was requested. Despite the efforts of all the professionals dealing with Peter, his behaviour had deteriorated beyond acceptable limits.

While at this point the powers of the probation order were formally subsumed by mental health legislation, no such mandatory demarcation was ever really experienced since the probation service and all other agencies remained involved and attended relevant meetings and their individual agency functions became parts of a greater and more coherent whole.

In September, the third risk management meeting negotiated the following plan.

- All agencies would continue to support the ward staff in their work with Peter.
- Police and social services would be informed by the psychiatrist of any plan for discharge.
- The probation officer and police officer would provide full offence material for the regional secure unit to aid the assessment process.
- The community care assessment officer would track the case, as future services might be required when assessment was complete.
- The consultant psychiatrist at the regional secure unit would be sent a copy of the risk management plan.

Discussion

It was necessary to formulate a shared opinion of the nature of the risk Peter presented. While this was to a degree speculative because of the nature of his mental health, it seemed inappropriate to define him as high risk without structured reasons for doing so. But each agency agreed, based on their general experience and skills in and approach to case management, that the mental health concerns surrounding Peter created unpredictability, so aggravating the risk of aggression to a level unacceptable to and unmanageable in the community. Had Peter been in good mental health, his offences would in themselves have caused sufficient concern to place him at high risk; his illness compounded this risk. Professional liaison worked well, and the risk management meetings were able to expand the focus of discussion from exclusively looking at the mental health problems to examining the potential for offending and attempting to address the relation between the two.

This demonstrated a commitment to SORMA which gave a positive message to all agencies. Scope for conflict existed but only very occasionally did it surface – notably and briefly when the first psychiatrist appeared not to be listening to the concerns being expressed by the other agencies, and was successfully persuaded, in the face of overwhelming pressure from others present, to re-consider the relationship between patient confidentiality and his public protection responsibilities.

Once an agreed level of risk was determined, it was agreed that libido-suppressant medication would provide an additional method of control, and it was disappointing that this had to be discontinued. It also became clear from the immense value of using the landlady as community collaborator just how unfortunate it was that no person had initially been identified to fill this position. The widespread use of such collaborators had proved particularly useful in the cases of other SORMA subjects, creating as they did a network of informants able to report risky situations as they arose, and to trigger an immediate and urgent professional response.

SORMA was implemented in the case of Peter with positive results. Multi-agency collaboration gave greater insight and direction in particular to the psychiatric management of a case which would otherwise have operated largely along therapeutic lines, so lacking the additional public protection neces-sary in the case of a potentially dangerous mentally disordered sex offender. Surveillance had led to concern that ultimately triggered the recognition of the need to use legislative authority to control the risk he presented, and only the multi-disciplinarity of the professional forum created by SORMA's risk manage-ment meeting system enabled the interaction between mental disorder and sex offending to be addressed in a way which ensured the support of a wide range of professionals, from police to psychiatrists, probation officers to psychiatric nurses.

As an afterword it can be added that, following a six-month assessment period at the regional secure unit, a case review was held. At this review, it was stated that Peter was a potential rapist and murderer, as a result of which he is currently detained on a long-term Mental Health Act section order. Though one can never know, it is not unrealistic to speculate that Peter's timely admission to the psychiatric unit may have prevented the rape and murder of a child; and that admission came as a direct result of the multi-agency collaborative framework created as part of SORMA.

Conclusion

Sex crime is the concern of many organisations both within and outside the criminal justice system. What is becoming increasingly clear is, first, that behind the individual functions of these separate organisations lies the common aim of public protection; second, that the extent of public concern with crimes of this nature is intense; and third, that the level of public, press and political demand that professionals offer effective protection is high.

Protection and prevention are therefore fundamental aims, universally recognised by the professionals involved. Multi-agency risk management provides a script written in universal language. It recognises the similarities in the duties of the different agencies engaged in community supervision, elevates commonality over difference, offers solutions to arguments about method, and elevates the sharing of responsibility over inter-agency squabbling. Bringing together different agencies to discuss individual offenders, and recognising too that the offender himself and his family and community have a contribution to make, appear almost too obvious to require spelling out. Each agency stands to gain from such an initiative, no abdication of normal accountability is entailed, nor is there necessarily any resource commitment: indeed, joint assessment may produce considerable savings, as it can and should lead to the more accurate targeting of resources and the avoidance of duplication of effort with other agencies.

In brief, the aims of multi-agency risk management are to:

- *facilitate* a joint approach to crime prevention;
- *benefit* from sharing information;
- *promote* shared responsibility and accountability;
- *increase* public confidence;
- *reduce* fear of crime;
- *respect and maintain* each agency's individual contribution;
- *reduce* opportunities for offending;
- *increase* the likelihood of detection;
- *exploit* the full range of legislation to implement offender risk management plans.

Multi-agency case management of mentally disordered sex offenders primarily involves managing risk. Treatment of whatever kind offered to an offender in the community does not represent a comprehensive programme of supervision; surveillance of often dangerous offenders, so restricting their opportunities to commit further offences offers an additional element to case management and an opportunity for multi-agency collaboration. A helpful next step, however, would be for one of the agencies involved to take the lead in coordinating and developing a case management approach to the more effective supervision of mentally disordered sex offenders; and there is certainly a case to be made for probation's suitability for such a role to be considered by policy-makers. The evidence of the potential of this approach to increase public protection in a context in which it is barely conceivable that penal policy will not in the medium term again be seeking alternatives to custody for serious offenders, is overwhelming. At present, the gap between the capacity of the prison and that of community supervision to offer public security by incapacitating offenders seems unrealistically and undesirably wide, not least since all but the most serious prisoners will one day be at large again. The SORMA approach outlined in this chapter offers an achievable means of reducing the gap, and so of increasing the effectiveness of the control of mentally disordered sex offenders – and, of course, potentially many other offenders too – in the community.

References

Association of Chief Officers of Probation (1996) *Community Based Interventions with Sex Offenders Organised by the Probation Service: A Survey of Current Practice.* Wakefield, West Yorkshire ACOP.

Barker, M. and Beech, A. (1992) 'Sex Offender Treatment Programmes: a critical look at the cognitive-behavioural approach'. Paper delivered to the British Psychological Society Conference, Harrogate.

Barker, M. and Morgan, R. (1993) *Sex Offenders: A Framework for the Evaluation of Community-Based Treatment.* London: Home Office.

Beckett, R., Beech, A., Fisher., D and Fordham, A.S. (1994) *Community-Based Treatment for Sex Offenders: An Evaluation of Seven Treatment Programmes.* London: HMSO.

Clear, T. and O'Leary, V. (1983) *Controlling the Offender in the Community.* Lexington, MA: D.C. Heath.

Cohen, S. (1985) *Visions of Social Control: Crime, Punishment and Classification.* Cambridge: Polity Press.

Fisher, D. (1994) 'Adult sex offenders: who are they? Why and how do they do it?' In T. Morrison, M. Erooga and R.C. Beckett (eds) *Sexual Offending Against Children: Assessment and Treatment of Male Abusers.* London: Routledge.

Freund, K. (1990) 'Courtship disorder'. In W.L. Marshall, D.R. Lewis and H.E. Barbaree (eds) *Handbook of Sexual Assault: Issues, Theories and Treatment of the Offender.* New York: Plenum.

Goode, E. and Ben-Yehuda, N. (1994) *Moral Panics: The Social Construction of Deviance.* Cambridge, MA: Basil Blackwell.

Grant, D.L.(1998) 'Supervising sex offenders in the community: The Sex Offender Risk Management Approach (SORMA)'. Unpublished PhD thesis, the University of Hull.

Harris, R. (1992) *Crime, Criminal Justice and the Probation Service.* London: Routledge.

Home Office (1992a) *Three Year Plan for the Probation Service 1993–1996.* London: Home Office.

—— (1992b) *Supervision of Sex Offenders: A Probation Service Strategy Document.* London: Home Office.

Kemshall, H. (1996) *A Review of Research on the Assessment and Management of Risk and Dangerousness: Implications for Policy and Practice in the Probation Service.* London: HMSO.

Lacey, M., Pendleton, J. and Read, G. (1983) 'Supervision in the community – the "rightings of wrongs"'. *Justice of the Peace*147, 120–123.

Lemert, E.M. (1967) *Social Deviance, Social Problems and Social Control.* Englewood Cliffs, NJ: Prentice-Hall.

McGuire, J. (ed.) (1995) *What Works: Reducing Re-offending: Guidelines from Research and Practice.* London: Wiley.

McGuire, J. and Priestley, P. (1995) 'Reviewing "what works": past, present and future'. In J. McGuire (ed.) *What Works: reducing Re-offending: Guidelines from Research and Practice*. London: Wiley.

McWilliams, W. (1986) 'The English probation service and the diagnostic ideal'. *Howard Journal of Criminal Justice*. 25 (4), 241–60.

Mair, G. (1996) 'Developments in probation in England and Wales'. In G. McIvor (ed.) *Working with Offenders*. London: Jessica Kingsley.

Mankoff, M. (1971) 'Societal reaction and career deviance: a critical analysis'. *The Sociological Quarterly* 12 (3). 204–18.

May, T. (1991) *Probation: Politics, Policy and Practice*. Milton Keynes: Open University Press.

May, T. and Vass, A.A. (eds) (1996) *Working with Offenders: Issues, Contexts and Outcomes*. London: Sage.

Pithouse, A. (1987) *Social Work: The Social Organisation of an Invisible Trade*. Aldershot: Gower Press.

Prins, H.A. (1986) *Dangerous Behaviour, the Law and Mental Disorder*. London: Tavistock Publications.

—— (1995) *Offenders, Deviants or Patients?* London: Routledge.

Raynor, P. (1996) 'Evaluating Probation: the rehabilitation of effectiveness'. In T. May and A.A. Vass (eds) *Working with Offenders: Issues, Contexts and Outcomes*. London: Sage.

Richardson, J.T., Best, J. and Bromley, D. (eds) (1991) *The Satanism Scare*. New York: Aldine de Gruyter.

Roberts, C. (1995) 'Effective practice and service delivery'. In J. McGuire (ed.) *What Works: Reducing Re-offending: Guidelines from Research and Practice*. London: Wiley.

Vass, A.A. (1982) 'The probation service in a state of turmoil'. *Justice of the Peace* 146, 788–793.

Young, J. (1971) 'The role of the police as amplifiers of deviancy, negotiators of reality and translators of fantasy: some consequences of our present system of drug control as seen in Notting Hill'. In S. Cohen (ed.) *Images of Deviance*. Harmondsworth: Penguin Books.

—— (1994) 'Incessant chatter: recent paradigms in criminology'. In M. Maguire, R. Morgan and R. Reiner (eds) *The Oxford Handbook of Criminology*. Oxford: Clarendon Press.

Chapter 7

The Parole Board and the mentally disordered offender

Judith Pitchers

Parole and risk: a new emphasis

The Parole Board of England and Wales advises the Home Secretary on the release on licence of determinate and life sentenced prisoners, on the recall to prison of anyone so released coming to adverse notice whilst they are on licence, and on any other matters referred to it (Section 32, Criminal Justice Act 1991). Since the Board was originally established by the Criminal Justice Act of 1967, the parole system in the United Kingdom has been subject to occasional intervention by Home Secretaries, and even to radical alteration by statute, most recently in the 1991 Criminal Justice Act. The overall effect of earlier changes had been a gradual shift in the balance of power towards Ministers and away from the Board, but the 1991 Act reversed this trend by scrapping the restrictive guidelines introduced by the then Home Secretary, Leon Brittain, which had severely limited the power of the Board to grant parole to long termers. The Act also increased the Board's executive powers, making it wholly responsible for releasing discretionary lifers and prisoners serving from four to seven years. The Board continues to act as an advisory body in relation to the release of very long-term prisoners and mandatory life sentence prisoners.

Despite the changes since 1967, parole has remained in essence a procedure whereby inmates are selected for early release on condition that they accept supervision by a probation officer and understand that they are at risk of re-call to prison to complete the balance of their sentence if they reoffend or otherwise breach their licence conditions (West 1972). The primary task of the Board is of course to decide which particular prisoners will be selected for early release, so that they may serve the remainder of their sentences in the community. In fact, the Board became an Executive Non-Departmental Public Body in 1996, but despite this and the changes enacted in the 1991 CJA, it does not have complete freedom to determine its policy or procedures and remains bound by broad policy directions issued by the Home Secretary. The directions currently in force were issued by Michael Howard under S.32(6) of the CJA 1991, and they instruct the Board, when making its deliberations, to 'consider *primarily* the risk to the public of a further offence being committed at a time when the prisoner would otherwise be in prison and whether any such risk is acceptable'. The directions go on to call upon the Board to consider whether

a. The longer period of supervision that parole would provide is likely to reduce the risk of further imprisonable offences being committed. In assessing the risk to the community, a small risk of violent offending is to be treated as more serious than a larger risk of non-violent offending.
b. The offender has shown by his attitude and behaviour in custody that he is willing to address his offending and has made positive efforts and progress in doing so.
c. The resettlement plan will help secure the offender's rehabilitation.

These explicit criteria replace a list of reasons for refusing parole, one of which was 'medical considerations', and thus seem to shift the parole decision away from a position of tacit acknowledgement that parole would be granted unless a good reason existed for refusing it. As the Board is called upon to 'consider' the criteria rather than be satisfied about them, these instructions could be construed as conferring a neutral stance towards the granting of parole. However, some believe that the wording of the new directions indicates that the Board is expected to take a more negative attitude than before, and that there is now actually a presumption that parole is to be refused unless the criteria are met (Hood and Shute 1995).

In any event, the directions make it clear that risk of reoffending, especially of violent reoffending, is now the primary factor in determining release. The procedures for the release of life sentenced prisoners differ markedly from that of determinates (i.e. prisoners given sentences of a fixed period of years), but the release criteria are similarly risk-focused. Indeed, once a life sentenced prisoner's tariff (the minimum period necessary for the purposes of deterrence and retribution) has expired, the only factor for the Board to consider when advising or directing release is that of risk to the public. The wording of the Home Secretary's directions on the release of mandatory life sentence prisoners is as follows:

> The Parole Board's responsibilities in the release consideration are whether, having regard to the degree of risk involved of the lifer committing further imprisonable offences after release, it remains necessary for the protection of the public for the lifer to be confined.
>
> (Home Office 1992)

Board members consider parole applications in panels of three. When the panels meet in London, their decisions are based solely on the papers put before them; at oral hearings conducted in prisons (for discretionary lifers and prisoners serving sentences at Her Majesty's Pleasure) the Board has the benefit of both documentary and oral evidence. In arriving at its conclusions, the Board may either be regarded as carrying out quite complex risk assessments of its own, or as simply accepting or rejecting the risks as assessed by others. Decisions and recommendations are based, at least in part, on multi-disciplinary risk assessments carried out on the prisoner during his or her sentence (Crighton, 1997). Until very recently the Board also had before it, when dealing with determinate sentence prisoners, the Risk of Reconviction (RoR) score, a statistical risk predictor designed for the Board's use (Copas *et al.* 1996). At the time of writing, however, financial considerations have (not for the first time) brought about the temporary suspension of the use of the RoR in order to save the cost of calculating the scores. Although the Board is thus deprived of an apparently useful tool in risk assessment, in practice the effect of this measure is unlikely to be great. Evidence suggests that RoR scores tend to be used to confirm decisions rather than to inform them, and may be disregarded where Board members consider that other factors indicate that the true risk differs substantially from the purely statistical (Hood and Shute 1995).

Risk and the mentally disordered offender

The new emphasis on the risk of violence could be expected to have consequences for the mentally disordered, since they are often regarded as particularly risky, or at least unpredictable. The RoR score did not incorporate the prisoner's psychiatric history, and at present there seems little prospect of finding a reliable, consistent and accurate actuarial risk predictor which takes into account 'dynamic' variables such as mental illness, instead of the purely static factors used by this predictor (Ditchfield 1997). However, the Training Guidance for Board members which accompanies the Home Secretary's directions lists 'any medical or psychiatric considerations' among the factors that the Board is to take into account when arriving at its decisions, and also suggests that the Board should have regard to any medical reports prepared for the court. Training Guidance on the release or transfer to open conditions of mandatory lifers goes a little further: the Board is to take into account any medical, psychiatric or psychological considerations (particularly where there is a history of mental instability). The Board is further directed to have regard to psychiatric reports when considering recall of all types of prisoners.

As other contributors to this collection have noted, the prison population contains a substantial proportion of prisoners who are mentally disordered or who have a psychiatric history; a survey of sentenced prisoners disclosed that 37 per cent of the sample had disorders that the researching psychiatrists could diagnose (Webster and Eaves 1995). More recently, Brooke *et al.* (1996) found that 63 per cent of the remand population were mentally disordered. Clearly, the existence of a psychiatric disorder may have a bearing on all three of the new criteria for release listed above. First, the diagnosis may be seen as *per se* increasing the chances of behaving violently while on parole licence. Second, ill or personality disordered prisoners may not find it easy to address their offending. This may be because of limited capacity to develop insight into the causes and consequences of their offending, or because erratic prison behaviour, dependence on medication, or general mental fragility debars them from attending cognitive-behavioural groups in prison. Attendance at these groups is one of the commonest ways for prisoners to show that they have 'made positive efforts and progress towards addressing their offending behaviour' (Home Office 1992: 3–4). Finally, it may be difficult for the mentally disordered person to establish an acceptable re-settlement plan, since families and hostels are often reluctant to take responsibility for them. Even when it *is* possible to make definite release plans, a mental disorder may be seen as such a fundamentally destabilising factor that it could fatally undermine the potential parolee.

In fact the difficulty of predicting criminality among the mentally disordered has long been acknowledged (Prins 1986 and 1990). Although mental disorder is also only weakly associated with violence – Webster and Eaves (1995) give an overview of the literature – this association has been observed to be constant. While there is a danger of overstating the link between most forms of mental illness and a propensity towards violent conduct, a stronger link can be shown where the offender is actively psychotic, or else is suffering from a serious personality disorder (Prins 1990). Psychopathy, is after all, legally defined in terms of abnormal aggressive and irresponsible behaviour (Peay 1997).

It is now well established that clinicians have a tendency to over-predict violent behaviour, resulting in many 'false-positive' predictions. However, Webster and Eaves (1995) point out that more recent research has tended to show a relatively high level of violent conduct among those mentally disordered persons for whom violence has been predicted, especially among patients suffering from personality disorders, and notably among men (women's violence was generally under-predicted). This suggests that clinical risk assessments may be more valuable than has traditionally been supposed.

If prisoners with a record of dangerous and unusual behaviour require detailed clinical assessments in order to establish the risk of re-offending (Ditchfield 1997), it is obviously important for these assessments to be provided for the Board. The parole dossier may include clinical opinions, or the Board may adjourn proceedings for their production when it considers that it is impossible to assess risk in their absence. However, the implications of such deferrals, both in terms of costs and delays, cannot be disregarded, and this step is not taken lightly or very often. It is more common for the Board, when refusing parole, to ask that a psychiatric report be produced at the time of the next review. Sometimes a report prepared by an independent consultant forensic psychiatrist is specified. Although the Board does not have the power to insist on the production of psychiatric reports, requests of this sort are usually honoured by the prison service.

Whether or not the dossier contains a psychiatric report, there may be a Board psychiatrist present to guide other members on the subject of clinical risk assessment. There is a legal requirement (currently under Schedule 5 of the CJA

1991) for the Board to 'include among its membership a registered medical practitioner who is a psychiatrist', and there has always been a percentage of psychiatrists serving on the Board – as at 31 March 1997, fourteen of the total membership of seventy-three were psychiatrists. The Parole Board has evidently been expected to rely on, or at least value, the clinical expertise that psychiatrists can contribute to risk assessment. This is a matter of Ministerial policy, and was most recently stated on 4 December 1997 (Hansard). All panels dealing with mandatory lifers include a psychiatrist, and there is always a psychiatrist member present at oral hearings, where it is common for the psychiatrist member to conduct sometimes detailed questioning of prisoners with a view to assessing their state of psychiatric health.

The Parole Board's policy towards the mentally ill

What special steps, if any, does the Board take to deal with the mentally disordered? In the first place, it is clear that the Board has not adopted any specific policy or attitude towards mentally disordered prisoners, nor do any of its key performance indicators (identified as part of the Board's Corporate Plan in 1996) refer to them. There is no requirement for non-psychiatrist members to be given specific training in this area, although new members' induction training and Annual Conferences often include discussion of psychiatric issues. The Board's *Policy and Procedures Manual* provides for the benefit of members an annexe giving brief working descriptions of the most common psychiatric disorders. Additionally, in recent years there has been specific training for all members on the risks posed by sex offenders, and Board Annual Reports disclose occasional visits by members to special hospitals and Regional Secure Units.

The lack of a stated policy is not necessarily a matter for concern. The Board's first objective, laid down in its Corporate Plan and agreed with the Minister and the Prison Service in 1996, is to deal with all cases in a consistent and equitable manner, taking into account any directions given by the Home Secretary. It may be argued that it would be wrong to adopt any specific policy towards the mentally disordered, or indeed towards any particular group of prisoners since every case should be considered equitably, consistently, and on its merits. But although it has no *policy* towards them, the Board has often drawn attention to the *problems* associated with dealing with the mentally ill. The Annual Report of 1987, commented, with reference to decisions where 'medical considerations' were a factor, that 'such cases can be very difficult', and more recently in its Annual Report of 1991 the Board stated that:

> we see cases in significant numbers who, judging from the reports prepared for parole, appear to be suffering from mental abnormalities . . . many display behaviour and thought processes which leave the Board in little doubt of their clear potential to commit further serious offences of escalating violence.

The report went on to say that the Board might recommend psychiatric assessment for such prisoners, and deplored the fact that no such assessment had been made earlier in their sentences. Regret was expressed that these prisoners had frequently to be refused parole on grounds of risk, with the result that they were released unsupervised when their sentences had been eventually served. This meant that the Board could do no more than delay exposing the public to risk from them.

Of course, following the 1991 CJA, prisoners who are refused parole are still subject to a statutory period of supervision when they are released at their 'non-parole date' (that is, after serving two-thirds of their sentence). It seems to be these particular prisoners, refused parole because of the risk they present, who now give grounds for special concern to the Board, which is responsible for determining any additional conditions to be imposed on the non-parole licences that lay down the conditions of supervision. The Board's 1994 Report drew attention to these problems, and to certain initiatives that it was taking in dealing with the mentally disordered.

> We have been increasingly troubled at the release of potentially violent prisoners with psychiatric problems . . . these prisoners sentenced to four years and over after 1 October 1992 have gone out into the community with probation support; and they have also benefitted from psychiatric oversight, hostel accommodation and offence-related programmes, when the Board has included these in the conditional release licence. Further, victims have been protected by 'no contact' conditions which forbid the prisoner to contact named people or return to named locations during the licence period . . . However, we have remained concerned not only about the high risk of offending posed by these prisoners, but about our own capacity to predict this risk and to identify the best way of accommodating these special needs. In 1994 we took three steps to address these problems.
>
> (Annual Report 1994: 4)

These steps were, first, the production of a Psychiatric Guidance note on risk assessment in reports for the Board, second, a new system of allocating cases to secure the input of a Board psychiatrist, and third, a tightening up of the procedures under which prisoners requiring psychiatric care were released.

Psychiatric reports for the Board

One of the problems faced by the Board is its lack of control over the quality and extent of any risk assessment, medical or otherwise, that has been carried out while the prisoner has been in custody, and which inform its own risk assessments. Many prisoners' dossiers contain no medical assessment at all, other than a brief negative response to the question 'Are there any medical or psychiatric factors (including dependencies) which may be relevant to consideration for early release on licence?' This question appears on the standard prison service form entitled *Medical Officer's Report to the Parole Board*, which is always part of the prisoner's dossier. Despite its title the form is not infrequently signed by someone other than a qualified doctor, probably a prison hospital grade officer, who may not even have proper nursing training. On occasions the assertion that there are no relevant medical or psychiatric factors relevant to parole appears to fly in the face of evidence elsewhere in the parole dossier. Sometimes the dossier includes a report from the prison doctor, who may or may not have a psychiatric qualification; in view of this a recent small-scale study of parole failures has suggested that prison medical officers should be 'dissuaded' from writing psychiatric reports (Barker 1998). The Board prefers to have reports from visiting psychiatrists, but the basis on which prisoners are selected by medical officers for psychiatric attention is not always clear. Furthermore, the length of the reports varies enormously from a couple of paragraphs to several pages, but they are rarely as comprehensive as pre-sentence or pre-trial reports. Reports on serving lifers with no psychiatric history may be more detailed than those on determinate sentence prisoners who *do* have a history of mental problems. Occasionally (indeed, frequently in the case of life sentenced prisoners), the dossier also includes a risk assessment from a prison psychologist, but such reports are relatively rarely prepared for determinate sentenced prisoners, other than sex offenders.

Because of dissatisfaction among Board members about the varying quality of psychiatric reports provided to them, in 1994 a note for the guidance of doctors writing psychiatric opinions for the Board was jointly written by a full-time Board member and a psychiatrist Board member. In early 1996, the guidance note was accepted by the Royal College of Psychiatrists and distributed by the prison medical service. The note, which specifically asks report writers to have regard to the prisoner's psychiatric history, both during this sentence and before it, continues:

> To assist the Board in assessing risk and framing any necessary licence conditions, please answer the following questions:
>
> 1. If the inmate is demonstrating bizarre behaviour or disturbance of mood, cognition or belief – and if you believe this to be the consequence of functional or organic psychiatric disorder – is there any pre-release treatment you can recommend and arrange? Does he/she have severe learning difficulties? If the inmate's condition is untreatable, does it preclude parole by elevating the risk of reoffending?
>
> 2. Can the inmate's mental disorder be treated post-release by drugs or cognitive behaviour or some other form of therapy? Can you recommend a specific psychiatrist, hospital or outpatient clinic to take on clinical responsibility for the prisoner upon release? (See below, in the discussion of post-release licence conditions, for the further information requested here.)

3. Does the inmate display an attitude either towards his offence, his history of offending or therapeutic programmes, which indicates probable lack of co-operation during a licence period? (Even if his problem is treatable, he will not benefit from parole if he is hostile to examining his offending behaviour or submitting to treatment.)

These parts of the guidance note are quoted nearly in full in order to demonstrate the detailed nature of the advice being given and the sort of answers being elicited by the Board to assist it in its deliberations, especially with regard to risk assessment and the framing of licence conditions. It is perhaps worth noting that to date, no study has been undertaken to assess the impact, if any, of the guidance note, or to monitor the quality of psychiatric reports now coming before the Board. Whatever the disquiet about psychiatrists' reports, there appears to have been little recent criticism from the Board on the quality of those prepared by *psychologists*. This may be because psychological reports are usually prepared by prison service psychologists whose training prepares them to make detailed, parole-orientated risk assessments.

Allocation to psychiatric panels

The second procedural change made by the Board was an attempt to make more appropriate use of its psychiatrist members when dealing with determinate sentenced prisoners. As psychiatrist Board members are relatively few in number, it obviously makes sense to conserve their expertise (Hood and Shute 1994). In their pre-1991 CJA study, Hood and Shute had found that specialist Board members were usually outnumbered and often outvoted by independent members. They suggested that the Board should pay more attention to the balance of panel membership in order to make full use of specialist expertise in addressing the new risk-based criteria. This has not proved easy. The lifer population continues to grow, and the introduction of time-consuming oral hearings for some lifers, at which a psychiatrist is invariably one of the panel, has resulted in greater pressure on psychiatrist Board members. Furthermore, in 1992 the number of Board members sitting on panels dealing with determinate cases was reduced from four to three, making it less likely that there would be a place for a psychiatrist member. In fact, in only about a third of determinate panels is there a psychiatrist present: in their later study, Hood and Shute found that independent members outnumbered 'experts' (a definition including judges, probation officers and criminologists as well as psychiatrists) in 67 per cent of panels they observed as against 44 per cent of the panels in their earlier study (Hood and Shute 1995).

Under the old system, determinate prisoners' cases were allocated to panels of the Board on the basis of the offence alone (for example, cases of those convicted of manslaughter on the basis of diminished responsibility, arson and sexual offences would automatically go to 'psychiatric' panels). This somewhat simplistic approach gave cause for concern, as it seemed to devote unmerited psychiatric consideration to some cases, and ignored many which would have benefited from a psychiatrist's expertise. To explore this hypothesis, four full-time members and the Board's fourteen psychiatrist members reviewed all cases allocated to psychiatric panels over a 3-month period, to identify those cases which required the expertise of a psychiatrist on the panel for a proper risk assessment. This exercise confirmed the hypothesis and led to the formulation of a check-list of criteria for inclusion into a psychiatric panel. Apart from those specifically deferred for consideration by a psychiatric panel, other cases deemed necessary for psychiatric assessment currently fall into three broad groups:

- Nature of the current offence: In these cases, the nature of the offence is sufficient to warrant psychiatric consideration. The offences are: manslaughter because of diminished responsibility; violent or sexual offences that are exceptionally savage or bizarre; arson except where the motive was financial gain.
- Psychiatric history: there should be a psychiatrist present where the Board is considering prisoners who have ever been diagnosed as suffering from mental disorder. The definition of disorder includes mental illness, mental impairment and psychopathic or severe personality disorder. Prisoners who have spent part of the current sentence in special hospitals, Regional Secure Units, or the 'therapeutic community' of Grendon Underwood Prison fall under this heading, as do prisoners currently or recently taking a range of drugs including major tranquillisers, anti-depressant, anti-psychotic and anti-libidinal drugs. Prisoners who have a recent history of self-harm or suicide attempts are referred to a psychiatric panel, as are those who display deteriorating violent or bizarre behaviour, and those whose dossiers include psychiatric or higher psychologists' reports which disclose mental health problems.
- Sex offenders: the Board considers that psychiatric expertise is necessary when considering certain sex offenders, that is those who, despite admitting their offences, have made limited progress on the Sex Offenders' Treatment Programme or refused to take part in it; prisoners admitting deviant fantasies; persistent offenders; and all paedophiles where the victim is under the age of 14.

It is clear that by no means all the prisoners selected under these criteria are or have been mentally disordered. The category covering prisoners with a psychiatric history is extremely broad; for example, having spent a period at Grendon is certainly not of itself a symptom of mental disorder, since the criterion for being allocated to Grendon is not mental disorder but a commitment by the prisoner to address the reasons for his offending behaviour. Sexual offenders against young children may have no previous history of similar offending, and no psychiatric diagnosis. The intention of the new policy was, however, to err on the side of caution and to try to ensure that all cases that could possibly benefit from a psychiatric input would be suitably allocated.

Psychiatric licence conditions

The third Board initiative concerned cases where it was deemed necessary to impose an additional 'psychiatric' condition on the licence of a parolee. This specific condition reads as follows: 'You must attend upon a duly qualified psychiatrist / psychologist / medical practitioner for such care, supervision or treatment as that practitioner recommends; (where known, the practitioner should be named, subject to their agreement).' It is obviously important that cases where a specific therapeutic need that can be met by the imposition of this condition are identified for the Board. Of course, in common with all extra-to-standard conditions, it can be imposed by the Board on a prisoner who has been refused parole but is being released at his non-parole date for a period on statutory licence.

The Board has no control over the management of risk in the community once the prisoner has been released, but it has now tightened the procedure for the imposition of psychiatric conditions. This change dates from a case in which a Local Review Committee, under the system operating before the 1991 CJA took effect, released a prisoner with a psychiatric condition although the supervising psychiatrist had not agreed to accept oversight, or even assessed his suitability for treatment. In the two-week period before such an assessment could be arranged, the man committed a very serious offence. Had the assessment been carried out while he remained in custody he might never have been released on parole; alternatively, had he been released under effective psychiatric supervision, those supervising him might have become aware of his deteriorating condition, and taken action to treat or recall him, thus preventing the offence. Although the Board was not responsible for release in this unfortunately notorious case, it drew the appropriate conclusions. There must now be a written agreement to accept guidance by the supervising doctor or psychologist before release, and failure to secure this may well result in a refusal of the parole application.

Prisoners transferred to hospital

Prisoners who because of acute mental disorder are transferred to hospital under S.47 of the Mental Health Act 1983, and subsequently recover before the expiry of their sentences, are usually returned to prison and dealt with in the normal way. The Board expects to be made aware of these cases, and information concerning transfers to and from hospital will normally be contained in the prisoner's parole dossier.

Determinate prisoners transferred to hospital during their sentences are not eligible for parole so long as they require treatment and remain in hospital, but the position of lifers is somewhat different. If it is believed that despite making a substantial recovery, the lifer would suffer a deterioration following a return to prison, a referral may be made to the Board while he or she remains in hospital. In July 1985 the Home Secretary announced that he would deal with mandatory lifers as if they had remained in prison and release them if so recommended by the

Board, and after consulting the judiciary. Oral hearings for discretionary lifers are also held in hospital if the patient is considered to be well enough. The Board judges risk in these cases on exactly the same basis as for lifers in prison establishments, and the numbers concerned are very low: one of the two lifers referred to the Board in 1995/6 was recommended for release, as was the only case referred to it in 1996/7 (Report of the Parole Board 1996/7). In *R v Secretary of State for the Home Department, ex parte Hickey and R v Secretary of State for the Home Department, ex parte H, F, B, and W* [1995] the Court of Appeal held that mandatory and discretionary lifers were not entitled to be referred to the Parole Board unless and until their medical treatment had ended or was no longer appropriate.

The Board occasionally has to deal with determinate prisoners whose dossiers seem to indicate that they could or should have been transferred to hospital before they became eligible for release, either on parole on at the non-parole date. Even if it appears that such prisoners will represent a wholly unacceptable risk to the community when they are released at their non-parole date, there is little that the Board can do. In exceptional cases, it is possible for the panel considering the case to write directly to the Prison Services Division, the Board's sponsoring body which acts on the minister's behalf, to alert them to the situation. In practice this will happen very rarely, and then only where there is very great concern about public safety, and the panel members believe that there is a need for urgent consideration to be given to the question of the prisoner's release. Of course information of this kind may come to the Prison Services Division from other sources.

Conclusion: risks to the public and risks to the rights of the mentally disordered

The parole decision balances the longer-term benefits of serving part of the sentence in the community against the risk of further offences being committed during that period. The new paroling criteria, which the Parole Board is bound to apply, place heavier emphasis on the risk of further offences than on the benefits of supervision. In any case, the Board will always seek to avoid releasing people who might commit serious offences while on parole, thus endangering the public and bringing the system into disrepute. Risks must of course be taken, because the only way to achieve nil risk would be to refuse parole to every applicant. However, in 1996, the Home Office Research and Statistics Department collated the results of parole research and concluded that during the first six months after release, fewer than 10 per cent of parolees offend, compared with 30 per cent of non-parolees. During two years post-release the comparable figures were 30 per cent as opposed to 55–60 per cent (Annual Report 1995/6). This may indicate that although Parole Board members arrive at their recommendations and decisions in a relatively unstructured and subjective way (Hood and Shute 1994 and 1995), they are nevertheless correctly selecting prisoners whose risk of offending is lower than average. However, it is difficult to be entirely confident in this conclusion, since it is impossible to determine to what extent other factors – particularly supervision and fear of return to prison – may be influencing parolees (Ditchfield 1997).

Unfortunately, many mentally disordered prisoners, who might be especially likely to benefit from parole supervision and other forms of care or monitoring outside prison, are *not* regarded as presenting an acceptably low risk, and are therefore not selected for parole. Hood and Shute (1995) found that the use of the new criteria had adversely affected the chances of prisoners perceived by the Board as high-risk: 33 per cent of such prisoners were recommended for release at the time of their final review, as opposed to 63 per cent in their earlier (1994) study. The introduction of statutory supervision for those sentenced after 1 October 1992 is also likely to have diminished the chances of high-risk prisoners being granted parole, since it can no longer be argued that they need a short 'launch', that is a short period on parole supervision, to assist resettlement into the community. The statutory period of supervision, following release at the two-thirds point, provides all non-paroled prisoners with a form of launch, something which may go some way towards meeting their needs in the period immediately after release. In general, then, the Board no longer needs to weigh the possible benefits of giving very high-risk prisoners a few months of supervision against the real risk of an immediate return to offending.

Hood and Shute (1995) regard the reduction in the number of panel members considering the cases of determinate sentenced prisoners as having had a radical effect on the Board's ability to function as a multi-disciplinary body. Immediately after it was established in 1967, the Board would sit in panels of five or six, so that all the five categories of members (independent, psychiatrist, judge, criminologist and probation officer) could be represented. By 1992 this practice had long ceased, with all panels comprising four members only. Following the implementation of the 1991 CJA and further reduction to three members for determinate cases, it became even more common for independent members to dominate panels (Hood and Shute 1995). A very recent development (Hansard, 4 December 1997) means that lifer panels are now also restricted to three members. In a three-member panel, the majority view always prevails. The inference may be that psychiatrist members have less influence than before, but no research has been carried out to determine the weight given to the views of psychiatrists by their fellow members. Certainly, Hood and Shute's research studies did not suggest that psychiatrists were pre-eminent in discussion or decision-making. It seems that the Board accepts the value of clinical, lay and actuarial risk assessments, and then arrives at its decisions by weighing these various assessments together with other factors that emerge from the papers and discussion of the case. In any event, there is no evidence to suggest that the decisions of panels where non-specialist members predominate are qualitatively different from decisions taken by other panels; research in this area would be very difficult and not surprisingly, none has been undertaken.

In the spirit of the new focus on risk, the Board has taken a number of steps in the last three or four years to try to improve the quality of its assessments of mentally disordered prisoners, and to assist the risk management of licensees. In particular, the Board has shown itself to be concerned about mentally disordered prisoners whom they consider to present too high a risk to be recommended for parole, but who of course have to be released when they reach their non-parole date. Judged by its occasional pronouncements and recent procedural initiatives, the Board seems tacitly to have accepted that the mentally disordered may be more prone to violent re-offending than other released prisoners, although it is unclear whether this judgement has been founded on the basis of research, risk assessments in the dossiers, or simply accepted conventional wisdom. Recent high-profile cases in which patients released from mental hospitals into the community have gone on to commit serious acts of violence will no doubt have influenced Board thinking. Members cannot but be aware of the damage that is inflicted on public confidence in the parole system when parolees commit serious offences, and they may well conclude that it is better to err on the side of caution when making risk decisions. Unfortunately, any move in the direction of caution is likely to result in more false-positive predictions. We know that the links between mental disorder and crime are frequently brought to public notice and exaggerated, and that it is easy for professionals as well as lay people to over-emphasise them (Webster and Eaves 1995). Most of the mentally ill are not violent or dangerous; but on the other hand, recent research has confirmed the relationship between the psychopathic or personality disordered and violence. Because of this, it is essential to maintain the distinction between these and other mentally ill prisoners whose propensity to violence may not be any greater than those without any psychiatric history at all.

Parole decisions are rarely based on one factor alone, and the majority of factors that affect clinical risk assessment influence non-clinical judgments also. The adoption of a policy to isolate mentally disordered offenders and treat them as a separate category for the purposes of parole would have distinct dangers, foremost among which would be that they would come to be seen by Parole Board members as automatically falling into a high-risk bracket. In fact, we have no evidence to suggest that the Board is moving towards adopting such a policy. There is, after all, no general agreement over what constitutes a mentally disordered offender in the first place (Peay 1997), a difficulty as relevant in parole decisions as in any other aspect of the criminal justice system. Of course, where prisoners have a psychiatric history, the Board needs to be fully informed of their current mental state, and the relevance of their condition, if any, to their chances of successfully completing parole. To this end, it is obviously sensible for the Board to continue to press for improvement in those areas where its ability to produce good risk assessments is dependent on other agencies. First, psychiatric reports must be provided where necessary, and the quality of these reports and other risk assessments should be monitored. Second, the probation service and other agencies should be encouraged to produce realistic and supportive release plans for mentally disordered prisoners, without which parole may be seen to present too many risks both to the offender and the community at large. As far as its *own* performance is concerned, the Board should continue to focus on making the best use of its members' psychiatric expertise. Given the large numbers of mentally disturbed prisoners in the long-term prison population, Board members who are not psychiatrists would probably benefit from more specific training in the area of mental disorders, and they should at the same time be made aware of research into the links between mental disorder and violent offending. It goes without saying that any changes in the Board's policy or practice ought to be based on this research and other evidence, rather than on generalisations about the nature of mental illness.

The duty of Board members is as we have seen primarily to have regard to risks posed by dangerous offenders, which means that such risks may often be judged to outweigh any benefits of supervision to the mentally disordered parolee. However, the duty of the Board not to expose the public to unacceptable risks, and the understandable desire to preserve the parole scheme from public criticism must continue to be carefully balanced against the risk of injustice towards the mentally disordered.

References

Barker, A. (1998) 'Parole failure study'. *Prison Service Journal* 115, Jan., 34–36.

Brooke, D., Taylor, C., Gunn, J. and Maden, A. (1996) 'Point prevalence of mental disorder in unconvicted male prisoners in England and Wales'. *British Medical Journal* 313, 1524–1527

Copas, J.B., Marshall, P. and Tarling, R. (1996) *Predicting Re-offending for Discretionary Conditional Release*. Home Office Research Study 150, London: HMSO.

Crighton, S. (1997) 'Risk assessment in the prison service'. *Prison Service Journal* 113, 2–4.

Ditchfield J. (1997) 'Actuarial prediction and risk assessment'. *Prison Service Journal* 113, 8–13.

Hansard (1997) 4 December, cols 295–6, London: HMSO.

Home Office Circular (1992) 85/1992, Annexe A: *Directions to the Parole Board under S.32 (6) of the CJA 1991*.

Hood, R. and Shute, S. (1994) *Parole in Transition*. Occasional Paper No.13, Oxford: University of Oxford Centre for Criminological Research.

—— (1995) *Paroling with the New Criteria*. Occasional Paper No.16, Oxford: University of Oxford Centre for Criminological Research.

Parole Board (1987) *Annual Report 1987*. London: HMSO.

—— (1991) *Annual Report 1991*. London: HMSO.

—— (1994) *Annual Report 1994*. London: HMSO.

—— (1995) *Annual Report 1995 and 1995/6*. London: HMSO.

—— (1996) *Annual Report 1996/7*. London: HMSO.

—— (nd) *Annual Plan 1996/7* (unpublished).

—— (nd) *Corporate Plan 1996* (unpublished).

—— (nd) *Policy and Procedures Manual* (unpublished).

—— (nd) *Psychiatric Reports for the Parole Board* (Guidance for Psychiatrists) (unpublished)

Peay, J. (1997) 'Mentally disordered offenders', In M. Maguire, R. Morgan, and R. Reiner (eds) *The Oxford Handbook of Criminology*. Oxford, Oxford University Press.

Prins H. (1986) *Dangerous Behaviour, The Law, and Mental Disorder*, London: Tavistock.

—— (1990) 'Mental abnormality and criminality – an uncertain relationship'. *Medicine Science and Law* 30 (2), 247–258.

Webster, C.D. and Eaves, D. (1995) *The HCR-20 Scheme (Version 1): The Assessment of Dangerousness and Risk*. British Colombia: Simon Fraser University.

West, D.J. (1972) *The Future of Parole*. London: Duckworth.

Chapter 8

Control and compassion

The uncertain role of Mental Health Review Tribunals in the management of the mentally ill

John Wood

Mental illness and legal restraint

The law and special legal procedures have been established to regulate the detention and control of those whose mental disorders give rise to fear for their own safety or for the safety of others. Because this control involves 'detention in hospital' or other serious curtailments of liberty it has to be both rigorously monitored and subject to challenge. There is at the same time an understandable belief that the judgement of relevant professionals – here largely psychiatrists and social workers – cannot be left to the standards of the individuals themselves, backed up by the rules and vigilance of their own professional bodies. Indeed, professional self-regulation alone is unlikely to be regarded in modern times as adequate protection for an individual whose liberty has been seriously curtailed.

It is for these reasons that a considerable body of mental health legislation has arisen (currently the Mental Health Act 1983 and the Mental Health Tribunal Rules 1983), supplemented by regulations and the inevitable case law. Together, these form a complicated set of rules that seeks to control and supervise the detention or restriction of mentally ill patients which include, as an important safeguard the right to a periodic challenge. Bearing in mind some of the practices in the nineteenth and early twentieth centuries, some control was essential – and it had to be of a public nature since the attitude of relatives and friends of the mentally ill could not be relied upon as a routinely effective safeguard. To ensure an independent and effective challenge, a special system of Mental Health Review Tribunals was created by the Mental Health Act of 1959. Current legislation that has developed from this statute provides a more readily accessible and much more informal process than an appeal to the regular courts by way, for example, of the ancient writ of *Habeas Corpus*. There is a great deal of academic literature describing the work of the tribunals, particularly in examining their effectiveness from the point of view of the patient (see, for example, Peay 1983). Less attention has been given to the very important question as to the relationship between the professional judgement of psychiatrists and social workers and the pattern of law and practice of the tribunals. This is especially important, since the tribunals' work has given rise to a quite complicated framework aimed at the protection of patients. It has, incidentally given a key role to lawyers. *Quo Bono*?

There are clear and fundamental differences between the approaches of medicine and the law. The one tends towards an individualised and paternalistic 'caring', the other is founded on universal ethical concepts of liberty and rights. But both ethics and rights are difficult and often vague generalisations and so are hard to apply and often difficult to reconcile in individual cases. This is easily demonstrated – the power to enforce detention or serious restrictions may be advisable and sought by an experienced and caring psychiatrist and a specialist social worker on well-founded medical and social grounds, but if it is resisted by the patient as a serious and unnecessary limitation on freedom, some sound method of adjudication between the two views is essential. To this end, access is available to the regular courts, but the relevant law and particularly the procedure are too 'weighty' to serve as a regular and accessible method of review. It was for this reason that specialist bodies, the Mental Health Tribunals, were set up so that where the restraints are disputed, the differing viewpoints of the carers – doctor, social worker and usually the relatives – can be fully assessed and set alongside those of the patient, so that an authoritative decision can be taken.

These tribunals have not entirely displaced the earlier remedies available in the courts, but have become a very regularly used feature within the pattern of control of difficult patients. Their work has been the subject of many studies, some of which are most comprehensive and impressive (see Peay 1983). Less attention has been paid to their underlying role and to their effectiveness in the wider context of the treatment of the mentally ill. The work of the tribunals brings into sharp focus the clash of two justifiable but contradictory forces – paternalism which is based on human concern for those who are ill and which underlies much of the mental health legislation, and personal liberty which is firmly enshrined in the common law and is a crucial background to the statutory provisions that are concerned with the protection of the mentally ill as well as their control.

In attempting to keep those fundamental principles in balance the law has an exceptionally difficult role to perform. Central to its task is psychiatric medicine, which both in respect to diagnosis and to treatment has many uncertainties, and remains to some extent controversial. (see for example, Shorter 1997). Yet inevitably, it is psychiatric medicine which offers the core evidence upon which the tribunal has to reach its decisions.

The differing roles of psychiatry and law

Much in the practice of medicine is inevitably imprecise. In none of the specialities is this so true as in psychiatry which to a considerable extent lacks the ready assistance of the likes of broken bones and identifiable bacteria. What Thomas Szasz (1960) once famously referred to as 'The Myth of Mental Illness', remains undoubtedly controversial – indeed, debates about the nature and sometimes the very existence of mental illness continue. Even in the more 'secure' areas of medical practice, it is commonplace, where there is substantial doubt, for greater certainty to be sought by way of 'a second opinion'. Not surprisingly, in one of the conditions where doubt as to diagnosis is most likely to be challenged, namely mental disability, the consequent loss of liberty which may ensue involves greater cause for challenge and gives rise to a considerable number of difficult cases.

The concern for loss of liberty is age-old. Though the traditional right of challenge – the ancient prerogative *Writ of Habeas Corpus* – is still available, it has been supplemented by the creation of the system of appeals to the specially created Mental Health Review Tribunals. Indeed, they have become a recurring feature in the treatment of those patients whose illness has led to restraints on their freedom, their ready availability no doubt helped by legal aid which at least makes the process inexpensive for patients, whatever might be burden on the exchequer. This has brought legal regulation and challenge very close indeed to the day-to-day management of patients, and has led to the likelihood that each detained patient will ask for a review at a tribunal hearing of the grounds for the detention. This will inevitably entail a discussion of the work of the hospital in which the patient is being treated and in particular of the judgement of the Responsible Medical Officer, as the law grandly calls the patient's principal psychiatrist. It is important to note that the tribunal is only concerned with the matter of legal restraint and not with the question of treatment, though it is inevitable that this will be raised and discussed in the course of the proceedings.

It is now almost routine, therefore, that when an Order under the Mental Health Acts is imposed, it will be challenged by the patient. The emphasis given to civil liberties has led inevitably to an awareness of the right to challenge. Indeed, the law itself in certain situations provides for a reference to a tribunal, without the need for an application by the patient concerned. The composition of the tribunals reflects the underlying concept of safeguard, and indicates that the decision will involve the three strands of expertise underlying the control to which the mentally ill offender is subject. Central is the medical diagnosis, and so the tribunal psychiatrist is expected to conduct, before the hearing, an independent assessment of the patient in order to assist the tribunal on this aspect. Second, since the protection of the public is one of the underlying reasons for the Order, a full social assessment is also of great importance. Accordingly, the 'lay' member of the tribunal, who very often – but not necessarily – has social work expertise and experience, has an obvious importance in assisting the tribunal with this aspect of the assessment. Finally, there is the role of the legal president of each tribunal, which in practice is less focused, being concerned generally to ensure that the legal rules and regulations are followed and that the procedure has all the aspects usually subsumed in the term 'natural justice'.

It is worthwhile noting the steady growth in the number of tribunal reviews that are held each year, something which is shown in Table 8.1. The category of 'restricted cases' comprises those patients who have been formally charged with a crime and have been ordered to be detained in hospital – usually a secure hospital such as Broadmoor or Rampton. The underlying potential of continuing

Table 8.1 Number of tribunal reviews, 1986–96

Year	Applications	Non-restricted		Restricted	Total
		s.2	s.3		
1986	5,046	1,503	2,409	1,134	5,046
1990	7,650	2,684	3,628	1,338	7,650
1995	13,390	4,008	7,753	1,629	13,390
1996	14,913	4,145	9,016	1,752	14,913

Source: Mental Health Review Tribunals for England and Wales, Annual Report, 1996

danger has led, sensibly, to their being regarded as a special category to be carefully contained in a secure and therapeutic hospital.

As we have already seen, the diagnosis of mental illness or the other statutory incapacitates of mental impairment, severe mental impairment and psychopathic disorder set down in Section 1 of the Mental Health Act 1983 present far greater uncertainty than most medical conditions. This is especially so where the mental state is characterised as being within the particularly difficult statutory category of 'psychopathy', a condition which some commentators have even been prepared to deny exists. Given the contested nature of 'mental illness', it is obvious that a readily available right of challenge by a patient is likely to be exercised. Even a patient lacking insight will receive prompting to do so from a variety of sources – nurses, the hospital social workers and lawyers who have previously acted for the patient are all likely to ensure that the right is exercised. The availability of legal aid removes any financial obstacle to an appeal. Indeed, a pattern of regular tribunals was clearly envisaged by those who drafted the law, for the law itself provides for periodic review where the patient has not taken any initiative, suggesting that the protection of the patient's freedom is seen as important as the treatment itself.

The process of decision-making

One of the most important underlying features of the work of the Mental Health Tribunals is the interaction between the legal, medical and social aspects of the tasks they perform. The basic dynamics of the work of tribunals are conditioned by two principal influences – the nature of the legislative framework within which they operate and the interaction of the three different, but complementary patterns of expertise embodied in the tribunal itself – legal, medical (that is to say psychiatric), and social work. In view of the multiplicity of perspectives potentially bearing on the way the tribunals operate, it is important to examine their role and functioning in more detail. Another way of expressing the problems that are being considered is to ask to what extent should, and in practice does, each 'strand' play a part in the process of the review in its distinct phases of the hearing and the decision making.

The hearing

It is generally accepted that the tribunal hearing should be as informal as is consistent with a dignified and thorough examination of the issues involved. The patient's first contact with the tribunal will be when its psychiatrist, some time prior to the sitting, makes the examination, which will be reported to the tribunal. This is a statutory requirement, so that the tribunal has an up-to-date independent medical assessment around which it can marshal the other evidence it requires. On occasion, although by no means routinely, the patient will seek an independent medical opinion to put to the tribunal, most usually in the form of an additional written assessment.

There is no structure laid down for the conduct of the hearing and so provided it has regard to the rules of natural justice and to the obligations of fairness, the tribunal is able to mould its procedure to meet the individual circumstances of the particular case. This is essential, since the awareness and abilities of the patient can vary so widely, but it is perhaps surprising that no standard model has evolved. For example, fairness dictates that the patient, for whom the outcome is a principal concern, should be able to put before the tribunal whatever is felt to be important. The disability of patients may on occasion require very special consideration to be given to the most effective and unintrusive way of obtaining information from them. This has to be considered along with the essential evidence of others – notably the Responsible Medical Officer and the social worker concerned with the patient's case.

For centuries, important legal disputes, whether civil or criminal, were decided by judge and jury. It was accepted that the professional role of the lawyers involved, the judge and the advocates, was to delineate the rules, ensure that the facts were fully revealed and leave the decision, after clear summing up and guidance from the judge, to the jury. The jury, except in a small number of specialised cases, were 'lay men', chosen not for their expertise, but for their general and everyday experience and judgement. The judge would control, but not direct the proceedings, and when the evidence had been presented, the issues would be put clearly before the jury through the arguments 'for each party'. The final 'summing up' of the judge was aimed at clarity; it had to be scrupulously fair, and such guidance that was given, except on legal points, was in no sense binding. This adversarial pattern has been adopted by many of the more informal specialist tribunals, such as Industrial Tribunals and Rent Tribunals.

This is not the place to debate the merits of the adversarial system, but it is of central importance here to stress that the Mental Health Review Tribunal should be regarded, as its name clearly indicates, as a review and not an adversarial 'contest' in the robust Anglo-Saxon fashion. It is plain that it is the duty of the tribunal itself to ensure that a full and effective review takes place. It is not a 'neutral' body in the full sense that a court is – a point made absolutely clear by the seemingly ambiguous role of the tribunal psychiatrist, whose duty it is to inform the tribunal of the conclusions he has formed from the prior examination of the patient. Obviously, his findings will be openly discussed in the proceedings in order to allow comment, but his dual role is one that is not often found in the normal pattern of 'legal' decision making.

In everyday practice it cannot be expected that a procedure involving an often seriously mentally disturbed patient can follow a rigid pattern. The decisions on how to proceed can illustrate clearly the tensions that are present. A few examples should make this clear.

- Most central is who begins. There is little doubt that whether the case has arisen from an application by the patient or by reference under statute to ensure that a review occurs if the patient does not act, the procedure is for the patient's benefit. In civil cases (and no one should dare to suggest that the MHRT is in any way comparable to a criminal case), the plaintiff goes first. So should the patient in a tribunal, yet even such a fundamental point as this is not always fully accepted.
- The elucidation of evidence from all who appear to help the tribunal needs to be sensitive to their roles. The differing backgrounds of those attending demands considerable flexibility – close relatives, for example, have to feel that their often conflicting emotions are appreciated. The RMO will clearly be of greater assistance to the tribunal if the diagnosis and prognosis offered are intelligently considered, rather than formalistically challenged. The under-lying approach has to be flexible and should avoid both the stilted formula of a court – where verbal games tend to be played, and the unstructured case conference, which can easily lose coherence.
- The most dangerous legacy that the standard court procedure can bestow is the 'art of cross-examination' which is at the very essence of the adversarial approach and appears to be based on the hopeful assumption that if the right question is asked, 'all the weakness of the other side will be magically laid bare'. It is an enjoyable art, but none the less a pernicious process which is plainly unfair to the nervous, the uninitiated and the slow-witted. Happily, it is rarely found in review tribunals, where it is rightly replaced by a structured discussion of the key points with patient, RMO and other witnesses alike.
- There are many subtle traps. For example, although the evidence most central to the decision will usually be the opinion of the RMO, followed by that of the social worker, it is most important not to allow the way it is received to give the impression that the Tribunal is on the side of those detaining the patient.

The decision making

The underlying tensions that have just been discussed are also present when the tribunal turns to consider its decision. The law has recognised in the structure of the tribunal itself that there are three components underlying the decision. The existence and extent of the illness and its likely effect on conduct are for the medical member, who will have had wide practical experience. The impact of a return to society, and particularly the nature of the pressures that will be encountered are essential factors that lie especially within the competence of the 'lay' member, whether he or she be a qualified social worker or the type of socially aware lay person usually chosen to sit on tribunals. It will be the Legal President's role to ensure that legal imperatives arising from application of the rules to the case under consideration are complied with and to help to elucidate difficulties which may arise, as well as to ensure some orderliness in the procedure. Legal difficulties are rare, so the President usually finds their role consists in structuring the hearing and adding his or her own opinions to those of the members during the debate at the end of the case.

It is rare that the decision is a conventionally 'judicial' one. The tribunal is best compared to a jury – perhaps one of the special juries that were once used in commercial cases, where intimate knowledge of the background was thought to be important. Above all, it has been entrusted with the task of making a mature factual judgement within a fairly simple legal framework.

The Restricted Cases present a slightly different pattern, in that the patient has been before the criminal courts and sent, for an indefinite period, to a secure mental hospital. Such patients are entitled to a pattern of regular tribunals where there is both the power to discharge and the duty to report their opinion generally to the Home Secretary, who regards such reports as one of the many foundations upon which a later decision to discharge the Order may be taken.

In fact – and interestingly for the purposes of a general discussion of the role of mental Health Review Tribunals, this procedure has an importance in that it gives, more openly, a clearer duty on the tribunal to express an opinion as to the patient's progress and current state. This ensures that a continuous picture is built up and although most patients who are restricted rarely remain in hospital for very long periods, some do, and in all cases the addition of the thorough and careful assessment made by a tribunal to the case notes cannot but be of benefit. Although this happens in practice, such a report is not spelt out as one of the tasks of the tribunal.

The role of the tribunals re-examined

Underlying this chapter is an unease about the true purpose of the Mental Health Review Tribunal system, for until this is clear its work cannot be adequately assessed. The apparently simple answer – to allow the patient to challenge the need for formal detention – is certainly the kernel of the system but it does not fully describe what goes on in practice, nor reflect the underlying expectations. The proportion of patients whose Order is discharged is so small as to give the impression that the exercise itself is misconceived. Yet the continual use of the right to appeal to a tribunal is valued – and cannot just be attributed to the zeal of lawyer representatives who have now almost fully colonised the tribunals. It is probable that the majority of patients, even those with limited insight, value the opportunity to request an outside review and, although it might be said that their judgement of the advantages may be affected by their temporary disability, there are further advantages to be gained other than discharge of the Order. Relatives who attend hearings often indicate relief at hearing the progress of the illness being frankly discussed in a sensitive but dispassionate way. Tribunal members no doubt on occasion ask questions that the relatives feel constrained to raise.

The patient may generally be assumed to welcome an opportunity to put his or her views before an outside body, which will be seen to listen seriously to what is said. Although rarely granting the formal aim of the procedure – the discharge of the Order – the tribunal may well, in explaining its decision, reflect to the authorities some sympathy with the underlying problems that exist for the patient. To the cynic, the exercise is perhaps 'formalistic', merely underlying what was already known and expected. But it can be seen as one of those 'routine' exercises that give the applicant some status and the opportunity of putting a firmly held view – inevitably rejected in the hospital – which while perhaps unlikely to find favour with the tribunal, may lead at least to words of encouragement and possibly some modest suggestions which will be of benefit to the patient-applicant.

If this is accepted as a reasonable interpretation, it is important to look at the structure and availability of tribunals with these factors in mind, rather than merely the very narrow formal conception of the role of the tribunal as almost wholly concerned with the need for the statutory order. It follows that the functions of the tribunal are likely to be clearly understood as a general review and not merely a forensic contest as to the justification for the Order. There has been a tendency over recent years for this to be increasingly accepted both by consultants and carers, who appreciate that a calm and constructive look at progress by an outside body with multiple skills can be an advantage. This 'wider approach' needs to be recognised by the tribunals as something that will be most effective if attention is given to several aspects of the system.

The availability and purpose of tribunals

It is important that the hearings come at appropriate times for the patient. It is obvious that if they are too early, they will be relatively ineffective; if too long delayed, the protective aim of the legislation is not fulfilled and there is the possibility of a legitimate sense of injustice. These problems are already in evidence because the current pressure of a large number of applications is leading at times to unacceptably long delays in holding a tribunal, once a request has been made.

It is not the purpose of this chapter to put forward a detailed set of reforms, but it is nevertheless important to indicate some of the changes that might be considered. Where a patient is detained in hospital for the first time it is very important that the tribunal is held as soon as possible, in order to reassure the patient that reasons for the detention have been independently scrutinised. On the other hand, a patient who has already had to be formally detained on a previous occasion is likely to benefit most from a tribunal hearing coming after a somewhat longer period in hospital – say, after three or four weeks – so that the early effects of medication on the relapse can be properly assessed and taken into account. In such cases of resectioning it is most unlikely that a serious error has been made – indeed, such errors rarely occur in any event. Similarly, a restricted patient, lodged in hospital as a result of a judicial decision, is likely to remain there for some time and it is sensible that tribunal reviews are spaced at reasonable intervals. The current routine, where the patient is almost inevitably likely to spend many years in hospital, tends towards tribunals which have little or no impact. Mindful of this, we might propose that there is no reason why, as an additional, subsidiary function the tribunals should not play a constructive role in case management, such as allowing the tribunals themselves to have some input into the appropriate timing of a succession of tribunals, within, of course, a clear statutory pattern of maximum allowable 'gaps'.

Indeed, a great deal of thought is still required as to the 'real' role of the tribunal. The power to discharge, in its various forms is clear, but the impact that the hearing and the reasons given for the ultimate decision have on the way the patient is medically treated is very uncertain. In practice, the opinions of the members of the tribunal, incorporated in the reasons given for their decisions are afforded attention and respect. Their status is, however, ill-defined and it might be sensible to give some thought as to how the views of the tribunal might be given a more formal status – perhaps as a recognised 'second opinion', which it has to be said is how they are increasingly treated by the vast majority of RMOs already.

In restricted cases, these problems do not arise so clearly. It is expected that the tribunal will report to the Home Secretary on a wide range of matters beyond the crucial ones of mental state and dangerousness. Cases of mental breakdown, treated in hospital, do, however, pose a considerable number of underlying un-certainties as to the exact role of the tribunal. Its concern is largely the justification for the restraint of the order itself. A very wide range of other matters, which certainly concern the patient, fall strictly outside the tribunal's powers, although recommendations have become acceptable and usually welcome.

In appropriate cases, a discussion about medication, the hospital regime (particularly in respect to the way the patient's time is spent) about leave and so on, proves to be valuable although there are some underlying difficulties in this. There is an uncertainty as to how far the law formally permits what might be construed as intervention in these matters, bearing in mind its central concern being the continuing 'need' for the order in its present form. Nevertheless, wider discussions are inevitable and the earlier resentment that on occasion they used to give rise appears to have largely disappeared – indeed, detailed consideration of various factors is generally welcome. Although the vast majority of tribunal hearings cope with these uncertainties successfully, it might be wise to give some clearer indication of the importance of this aspect of their work.

Colonisation by lawyers at the hearing

There are two important underlying considerations here. The tribunal is reviewing restrictions imposed under statute and so, although the hearings are always concerned centrally with the mental state of the patient, the most important question is the underlying one of 'liberty'. Its loss has to be strictly justified in law, and so it is essential that the tribunal has appropriate legal knowledge, but above all it requires experience and judgement far wider than mere knowledge of the statutory rules themselves. The selection and weighing of evidence, even in formal court procedures involving a jury, require the initial guidance of a legal mind – hence the summing up by the judge. A similar task, this time informally performed, falls to Legal President of a tribunal. Yet beyond that a tendency for the Legal President to dominate has to be resisted.

That said, the crucial questions in a tribunal case are very wide-ranging and require consideration with a blend of professional expertise and worldly experience. The current mental state of the patient-applicant, the insight that the patient appears to have, the risks that removal of the Order may bring, the likely success of return to the community, and the extent to which there is support in the community are all essential to have assessed. It is the experience and judgement of each of the three members which are crucial at that stage and it is important that none predominates over the others. The technical, legal and medical questions apart, it is essential that the decision should be a corporate one.

One of the most subtle influences of traditional legal procedures arises in the form that the hearing takes. Television has made everyone aware of the dramatic, adversarial court procedure that is often taken as the norm for all 'legal' matters. Without doubt, the tribunal procedure should be structured rather than formal, and has to avoid rigidity without ever losing sight of its purpose. A tribunal which resembles a case conference lacks the degree of formality that such an important hearing warrants – equally, one which resembles a criminal trial is thoroughly insulting to the patient and can never be properly termed a 'review'. It is often difficult for the president of a tribunal to achieve an appropriate form for the hearing in a particular case. The varying abilities and disabilities of the patient make it unwise to consider a standard pattern as appropriate. There must be a conscious variation to meet the needs of particular patients and to take into account the representation of the patient by a lawyer, as is now usual. But certain crucial questions remain, and are rarely discussed. A few examples will be enough to show how important and difficult these matters can be.

• The question of 'Who shall begin?' has already been mentioned. As it is the patient's application, logic would indicate that the patient should, with the help of a lawyer, be asked to explain why he or she feels the time has come for the order to be removed. A fairly lengthy, wide-ranging conversation with the patient, with each member playing a part in order to assess the general abilities and above all the patient's insight into their illness is essential.

- There is the role of the patient's solicitor. It is wise to ensure that this is settled before the hearing begins. Generally speaking, common sense would indicate that the tribunal members each in turn talk to the patient and when this is completed the lawyer, or other representative, is asked to deal with any matters that it is felt has not been adequately covered. Again, although questions and answers are the inevitable form, they should not be used to pre-structure the hearing or to prevent anyone – patient or whosoever – from saying and particularly explaining things as naturally as possible. It is rare to find representatives, to whom the procedure is explained, who do not welcome a structured but informal type of procedure
- Other witnesses have a role. It would be tedious to consider in any detail the variations that are appropriate for each of these. The Responsible Medical Officer must obviously expect a rigorous examination of his opinions and a careful consideration of his plans for the patient. Nurses, who tend to know patients best, usually feel most at ease being allowed to say what they have already decided they would like to say. Their input is inevitably of real value. Parents and relatives cannot be expected to be detached and unemotional, and great care has to be taken not to force them to express opinions they clearly hold which they do not want to say openly in front of the patient. The approach of relatives is not so predictable as that of the professional carers, and does not fit easily into pre-determined patterns. It is important they feel that they have been able to say what they want to say, have not been badgered into saying things before the patient that may damage their relationship, and that above all they have had special consideration.

Put in general terms, a good hearing probably lies somewhere between the conventional court procedure and a well-conducted case conference. It is a brave and foolish person who would argue that there should be a standard pattern, although a clear framework is essential. It should result in a decision that is the result of combined deliberations, in which each has contributed, especially on those aspects on which their expertise and experience enable them to speak with added authority. The process is best regarded as a specialist jury function which should be guided but not dominated by the legal chairman.

Standardisation

The regional structure has many advantages. The nature of the work of the Mental Health Tribunals is intimate and benefits from clear local links. It does, however, lead to many variations in practice which, though not generally harmful in themselves, may indicate a lack of fundamental thinking as to the process of evaluating patients in the most effective way. It is a matter of taste whether some occasionally odd variations are preferable to rigid uniformity. There is, however, a subtle danger of the domination by the legal Chairman, towards which there is some evidence of a natural tendency. Although rightly chosen to preside over the

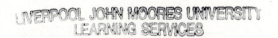

panel of three chiefly, but not solely, for specialist legal expertise – a logical approach, clarity of mind, the appreciation that all issues have two sides – lawyers tend to bring with them their own traditional preferences, particularly on procedure. It might be appropriate to indicate two particular assumptions most likely to affect the 'feel' of a tribunal hearing – an adversarial approach and undue formality.

The adversarial approach

Although there may be room for two opinions, it is very difficult indeed to accept fully the adversarial principle that all issues are best decided by assuming that there are only 'two sides'. It is certainly an approach that has to be modified in respect of the work of mental health tribunals. Obviously, the carers and the patient are seeking different outcomes from the proceedings – although it has to be noted that patients often apply for a tribunal hearing with no hope, or indeed desire, for the order to be removed. They seek to hear, in a reasonably formal setting, the reasons for the restraints and to put some contrary views that they hope will be considered by the tribunal and above all noted by those caring for them. It is surprising how often these aspects of a tribunal hearing have real substance. In those circumstances, the judicial function – deciding between two opposing and often over-stated views – is inappropriate.

Undue formality

The central questions to be decided by a Mental Health Tribunal are demanding. They have as two of their essential objectives the assessment of human personality and an estimation of future conduct. Both of these entail making judgements and inferences. This is more complex than the basic process of accurately finding facts and applying clear legal rules to them. The tribunal decision is fundamentally a human assessment, requiring experience and wisdom, and a recognition of fallibility. These are gifts enjoyed by many lawyers, but the structure of much legal practice and more especially the traditional court procedures do not encourage their use. In the traditional court, with judge and jury, the judge was expected to lean towards the calm elucidation of facts and the subsequent application of rules to them, while juries were the representatives of human experience and 'judgement', given the very difficult task of assessing the evidence for its worth, a task with an inevitably subjective element.

Conclusions

There are two very special features of the system of review that can never be overlooked. The first is that the holding of the review is itself an important indication to all concerned that the detention order is a very serious curtailment of liberty which must be carefully monitored. The monitoring has to be done regularly, and has been indicated above, ideally it should be undertaken at appropriate intervals. It has to have some impact, on both hospital and patient, otherwise in a large majority of cases and where the Order is very clearly essential, it has no purpose. Although the tribunal, rightly perhaps, has no legal power over matters other than the need for the Order, it is generally recognised that it is appropriate for it to give a careful assessment of progress. Indeed, on many occasions, its informal 'second opinion', modestly advanced, will be of assistance to an RMO who has some doubts about aspects of the patient's progress. Above all, the hearing and subsequent reasons for a decision are an excellent opportunity to indicate to the patient that progress, where it exists, has been acknowledged.

The second feature is that the process of review by a tribunal is a special type of intervention which should not mirror the adversarial structure of the normal civil, or more especially criminal courts. The dignity and formality that must obviously be accorded to an important matter are essential, but they should not be taken as requiring the standard procedures of a court, especially not a criminal court. The formality, their strict concern with relevancy, and the rigid elucidation of evidence by question and answer are some of the usual features of a court which have to be modified. There is, for example, everything to be said for a discussion with the patient on general, everyday matters, such as football or current events, and of the daily routine in hospital, so as to gain a wider understanding of the pressures and problems that the patient is likely to encounter in the community. It is even more important to ensure that the patient does not feel that he or she, rather than the statutory order, is 'on trial' at the hearing. There is a level between that of a formal court procedure and an unstructured case conference which appear most appropriate for the Mental Health Tribunal. Its exact form will vary according to the needs of each particular case. It has to be recognised that although there is at each hearing an underlying 'hard' question – should the Order remain in place? – there is a great deal more required in the task of reviewing the need for the Order.

There can be no other tribunal that is faced with such uncertainties and complexities as those of the Mental Health Review Tribunal. In most cases, the achievement of the tribunal lies beyond the mere decision as to the need for the Order under review. What is most appropriate, both for the patient and the community, differs in each case and is rarely easy to determine. Inevitably, the members realise the importance to patient, relatives and society of the impact of their decision. Similarly, those caring for the patient will very rarely have formed their own opinions except with deep thought, sound professional knowledge and much experience. Tribunal members are aware of the difficulty and importance of what they do, and never take their responsibilities lightly. It is important that they should be able to review Orders, at appropriate times and with as wide a choice of outcomes as possible.

Each case is a constant reminder that fate can be very cruel indeed. The system of Mental Health Review Tribunals is an appropriate recognition that society has to ensure, as far as possible, the provision of dedicated care for those whose mental illness gives rise to fears of dangerousness – to themselves or to others. Such care in a civilised society must endeavour to balance essential supervision, assistance and guidance, on the one hand, with as much freedom as possible, on the other.

References

Mental Health Review Tribunal for England and Wales (1996) *Annual Report 1996* London: Department of Health.

Peay, J. (1983) *Tribunals on Trial: A Study of Decision Making under the Mental Health Act.* Oxford: Oxford University Press

Shorter, E. (1997) *A History of Psychiatry: From the Era of the Asylum to the Age of Prozac.* New York: Wiley.

Szasz, T. (1960) 'The myth of mental illness'. *The American Psychologist* 15, 113–118.

Chapter 9

Thinking horses, not zebras

Jill Peay

The killing of Jonathan Zito by Christopher Clunis in December 1992 was a tragedy (Ritchie *et al.*, 1994). The nature of the killing was horrific; a former psychiatric patient stabbed a complete stranger three times in the head (once through the eye) on an underground station platform. It was a highly improbable occurrence.[1] Yet, the killing contributed in no small part to a re-evaluation of a series of complex and intertwined responsibilities and relationships; most notably, but not exclusively, those between patients and clinicians (Peay 1997). It is right that such a re-examination should have taken place and that it should have proceeded on two fronts; retrospectively, in respect of the circumstances surrounding homicides by those who have had contact with the mental health services (see Peay, 1996) and prospectively, in respect of what standard of care we can and should expect of those charged with some responsibility for the mentally disordered, once they have left hospital. One central paradox emerges; that we exaggerate with hindsight what we could have predicted with foresight (the 'inquiry' problem), yet we minimise the standards against which we will hold accountable those making judgements about what might happen (the 'negligence' problem). The consequence of the former has been that practitioners have felt demeaned and threatened by the potential for the attribution of failure by such inquiries,[2] while victims, secondary victims and patients have had their expectations of redress raised, and then dashed by civil actions for negligence which have come to nought when tested against the latter standard in the courts.[3]

In attempting to examine this paradox, this chapter seeks to identify itself with one pivotal theme in Herschel Prins's approach, namely, that difficult problems crossing disciplinary boundaries need to be informed by humanity and patience; in essence, his approach has been the antithesis of John Major's remarks about offending, that we need to 'condemn a little more and understand a little less'. Moreover, the chapter takes as one of its detailed points for examination an issue already explored by Herschel Prins (1996), to wit, the role of good communication in risk assessment and management. In short, this chapter is about how the realities and difficulties of the day-to-day care of the mentally disordered are thrown into stark relief by legal processes, and about how those processes may also ultimately impact negatively on that care.

Inquiries after homicide

As Crichton and Sheppard note, 1995 saw 'an explosion in the number of psychiatric inquiries, all focused on homicides committed by the mentally disordered' (1996: 65); these inquiries represented a marked shift in focus, from those which examined the abuse of power within mental hospitals, to a growing anxiety about the lack of control exercised over former patients at large in the community. At the same time, and as the impact of the NHS Executive Guidelines published in May 1994 became clear, attention shifted to the apparent frequency of homicides by the mentally disordered (Department of Health 1994); requiring an inquiry (which the guidelines now made mandatory) after every killing by a patient who had had contact with the mental health services was likely to lead, on average, to some 50 inquiries a year, not only generating an 'inquiry industry' but also heightening fears in the public's collective consciousness about the risk posed to their safety by the mentally ill. In turn, there have been repeated calls that lessons should be learnt from these inquiries, in order that such events might be prevented in future (Sheppard 1996). This is perhaps overly optimistic since, although the inquiries have made frequent criticisms of the events (and, more commonly omissions) leading up to a homicide, they have also largely concluded that the ultimate tragedy was neither predictable nor preventable. In this context, reducing the probability of such events is perhaps the best that can be hoped for.[4] None the less, the inquiries have created considerable momentum about the need for change, and have raised the expectations of secondary victims that there may be a basis on which they can seek redress for the errors of the professionals involved. Indeed, in a context wherein the care of the mentally ill has become highly politicised and the mentally ill demonised, it might cynically be argued that Inquiries after Homicide have been 'used' superficially to improve our understanding, but politically to shift the burden of responsibility from systems to individuals.[5]

But another consequence of these inquiries is also evident. Their retrospective approach, with its emphasis on the fine detail of the actions and omissions of those in contact with the mentally disordered perpetrator, leads to a highly subjective assessment of how 'failure' came about. The nature of the inquiries' recommendations (and when put together, they constitute a formidable list) then form a 'gold standard' of what might ideally be done in any future case (see Petch and Bradley 1997). The ways in which staff can fail to meet these standards have not only to do with the particulars of their own case, but also concern the multiplicity of recommendations made across the cases. Having cast the imperative in terms that we must all 'learn lessons', the inquiries encourage practitioners to adopt both the recommendations of the inquiry into their particular factual set and the general (and sometimes specific) recommendations of all other inquiries, thereby raising service standards across the board. Whether it is appropriate to cross-fertilise in this way is another matter. However, it is regrettable that if the inquiries' recommendations come to form the basis of what constitutes the acceptable standard of behaviour, such recommendations might never be set into the context of human successes and system failures.

Although the inquiry reports are not explicitly about blaming, nor do they largely attribute responsibility, they may: (a) be perceived as such by the subjects of the inquiry; (b) be regarded as such by secondary victims; (c) be used as such by politicians and the media; and (d) potentially be used as a baseline for ascribing negligence culpability. This latter problem is the prime concern of this chapter.

Actions for negligence

In marked contrast, the law's approach to the attribution of negligence is fundamentally prospective. Although litigation also proceeds on a case by case basis, the standard against which behaviour is judged is an objective one; what is it reasonable for the practitioner to do or foresee in the circumstances of the case? Although in the long term the range of inquiry recommendations may serve to enhance what can reasonably be expected, in the short term the courts test the breach of the duty against a relatively low threshold.

Indeed, the culture of blame reflected in the inquiry movement (Reder and Duncan 1996) – and the growing litigiousness which stems from it – is somewhat out of keeping with a system of tort law based on duties of care to 'neighbours'. Whether these are cast in the positive (love your neighbour as yourself); or the negative Rabbinic version formulated by Hillel (do not do to others what you do not want done to yourself), they imply a guide to ethical behaviour aimed at harm reduction, rather than the pursuit of maximum individual happiness or maximum individual redress (Reiner 1998).

The traditional starting place for our thinking about the approach of common law to negligence is Lord Atkin's statement in *Donoghue v Stevenson* [1932] AC 562. This required a man to avoid acts or omissions which he can reasonably foresee would be likely to injure his neighbour. The question then arises, who is a neighbour?; the answer comes (at AC 850) as 'persons who are so closely and directly affected by my act that I ought reasonably to have them in contemplation as being so affected when I am directing my mind to the acts or omissions which are called into question'. Neighbours thereby include cases both of those physically proximate and of those who are reasonably foreseeable; moreover, the plaintiff does not have to be individually identifiable by the defendant; it is sufficient that he or she forms part of a class of people whom the defendant should have in mind. But the fact that plaintiff is foreseeable does not mean that a duty will be held to exist, as a number of policy considerations serve to restrict or limit the extent of the duty of care.

The doctor/psychiatric – patient relationship has been embraced by this in a number of ways. The position in hospital is clear-cut; doctors owe both a common law duty of care and have various statutory duties under the Mental Health Act 1983. Moreover, where patients are inappropriately at liberty and harm themselves, for example attempting suicide, they can seek compensation for that harm against the relevant health authority. However, what is less clear is whether third parties injured by psychiatric patients (inappropriately) in the community can seek damages against the health authority.[6] Generally in English law, the courts have been very reluctant to impose a duty on one person for the torts committed by another (such third party liability does arise in other jurisdictions – most notoriously for mental health professionals in the USA following *Tarasoff*). This is not to say that it never happens,[7] for the courts have imposed a duty of care where the plaintiff has satisfied the court that the doctor's knowledge of the risk was sufficient to make it 'just and reasonable' to do so. However, *W v Egdell* [1990] 1 All ER 835 supports the proposition that such liability should be limited to cases where the threat was specific and was a threat of physical violence.

With the demise of the *Clunis* litigation, a new hurdle has been created, for although the difficulties of establishing third-party liability have been clear, the litigation had been proceeding on the basis that the health authority owed a duty of care to Clunis (the offender) while a patient in the community, for breach of which he could recover damages (partly for the prolonged detention he faces following his conviction for manslaughter). This would have been analogous to the attempted suicide situation above. However, the Court of Appeal, despite one authority to the contrary,[8] struck out the case on the bases that: (a) the plaintiff's claim was essentially based on his own illegal act of manslaughter; and (b) any alleged breach of the statutory duties should not give rise to a claim for damages (as the Mental Health Act provides an alternative remedy; namely enforcement by the Secretary State under S.124 where an authority is in default and/or judicial review) and it would not be just and reasonable to superimpose a common law duty where after-care was to be provided on a statutory basis.

Several interesting points arise which may make the decision vulnerable in respect of (b) above, and these are discussed below. However, one point in respect of the Clunis' wrongdoing is worthy of mention here. Stephen Irwin QC argued that Clunis' responsibility for the manslaughter had been significantly diminished and that therefore the maxim about plaintiffs not benefiting from their own wrongdoing should not apply. The Court rejected this, seemingly arguing that any degree of culpability would suffice. However, what would have happened had Clunis argued at his trial that he was not guilty by reason of insanity? No *criminal conviction* would have then resulted. It will remain an open question whether the long-perceived attractions of the diminished responsibility plea will be sustained where defendants like Clunis may be able to argue that they were M'Naughten-mad at the time of their offences.

However, even had the wreckage of the Clunis case not muddied the waters in respect of whether a duty exists, a substantial hurdle would still face plaintiffs; namely, to satisfy the duty the doctor only has to have acted in accordance with the practices of the reasonably competent member of the profession. Might that standard be vulnerable to being raised as a result of the multiplicity of recommendations made by inquiries?

And if the title of this chapter is not now evident, it derives from the notion that it may be more important to think about commonplace matters than to focus on the unusual.[9] For, seductive as it may be, the unusual can be misleading and potentially detrimental to the needs both of the mentally disordered and to the public's appreciation of their true position. The litigation surrounding the case of Clunis is one such example. Deriving from highly unusual facts, facts from which it must have been extraordinarily difficult for the Court of Appeal to distance themselves, Clunis may not only himself have been denied redress on policy grounds, but his action may also serve to count out for all time the claim that clinicians' responsibilities for their patients extend in a legally redressable form beyond the hospital into the community.[10]

Effective communication and the human condition

The Report of the Inquiry into the Treatment and Care of Raymond Sinclair is not atypical of the range of recent reports into 'Inquiries after Homicide' (Lingham *et al*. 1996). Sinclair fatally stabbed his mother in November 1994. It is difficult to summarise the complexity of his prior dealings with the mental health services, or do justice to the detail – of who said what to whom when – included in the Report. However, amongst the salient matters were his diagnosis of schizophrenia; the fact that he was abusing alcohol in the context of medication; that he had had a violent upbringing and was living, at the time of the homicide, in extremely poor accommodation with a family who expressed real concern about his behaviour – living in practice with a family who were in fear of him and fearful for him. Moreover, Sinclair had himself reported to his community psychiatric nurse thoughts of wanting to kill his mother and/or his brother. He also reported experiencing command hallucinations. These had led to a previous attempted stabbing of his brother just over two months prior to the fatal events. In short, Sinclair had all the tell-tale signs of being high on John Monahan's 'ladder of dangerousness' (Monahan 1993; 1996); with hindsight it is very easy to ask why the professionals had failed to put all these signals together and take appropriate action. However, it is worth digressing briefly into the detail of the Report in an attempt to understand the perspective of the various parties who 'failed' to act with sufficient urgency.

Ms Till was a basic-grade registered mental nurse with a diploma in counselling. She had no previous experience as a community psychiatric nurse. Raymond Sinclair was her first patient. She emerges remarkably well from the Report, exercising considerable skill in persuading him to be admitted to hospital after the attempted stabbing of his brother in August 1994. However, the incident was subsequently reconstructed by the patient as mere 'play-wrestling', and he was discharged only seven days later. This left Ms Till with the impression that the hospital team did not consider his condition as serious or life-threatening, in turn undermining her confidence in her own judgement (see para 4.5.2). When, on 1 November, he reported to her renewed thoughts of killing his mother (of which he said he was in control), she documented it and discussed it with his social worker, Ms Chater. But Ms Till did not telephone the consultant Dr Mikhail. Instead, she wrote to him on 2 November; tragically, the killing occurred on the 3rd.

Ms Chater, the social worker, who had recently been on holiday and sick leave, was unaware that Raymond Sinclair's brother had moved out of the flat they shared with their frail mother, leaving him alone with her. (There is a suggestion in the Report that the family may not have disclosed this information, as they wanted to maintain their priority status for re-housing.) Ms Chater's written observations, following a home visit after the attempted stabbing in August, were brief (para 4.4.7). However, she had been encouraged to be more concise in her reports and anyway, only a small space was available on the contact sheet for her to record the visit. The tension between summary information which loses important detail and detailed reports which swamp subsequent readers is commonplace.

Dr Mikhail, the responsible consultant, is described in the Report as having an excessive workload. In addition to his non-clinical commitments, he was based at three sites, where he was almost single-handedly responsible for acute care for a population of 110,000 – almost three times the case load recommended by the Royal College of Psychiatrists (para 3.3.5.) Dr Mikhail expected Ms Till to contact him if she were concerned; she thought he would take the initiative to inform himself if he were concerned.

Finally, there is the matter of Sinclair's case notes. On an earlier admission, following a ward round, Dr Mikhail (para 4.2.32) noted that the patient 'appears to be becoming dependent on hospital staff – goes home on leave and comes back with frivolous excuses'. This is, of course, curious from the perspective of Sinclair, who claimed that he had downplayed his symptoms because, like many patients, he did not want to stay in hospital. As the Report questions, did these repeated visits represent 'a perhaps not fully conscious attempt on his part to bring to the attention of staff the extent of his distress and psychosis' (para 4.2.32). Such ambivalence by patients is common – wanting out, wanting in – and is problematic for staff. However, once Dr Mikhail's observations were recorded in a comprehensive running note, they were there for all time and potentially could colour (arguably, authoritatively) any further appraisals.

Thus, the Report paints a picture of an under-resourced service and of inexperienced and inadequately supervised staff working under stress. A potent cocktail was clearly, with hindsight, in place. On the one hand, the records were too succinct to be useful, whilst others recorded detail which may have been misleading. The patient and his family were not only free agents, but may also have been motivated not fully to disclose everything that was going on. The constellation of professional carers were either overworked, or undermined and lacking in confidence, or not fully up-to-date with the minutiae of the patient's case.

Again, it is easy to make these observations with the benefit of hindsight; in prospect, identifying and recording what were the salient features would have been much more problematic. Yet, the methodology of the inquiry produces a picture which collates all the information which *could* have been known at any given time in a perfect world. Theirs is a retrospective, calm and thorough approach, but it may overplay the science of the possible in a world where the art of the improbable intermittently holds sway. Thus, the inquiry's methodology may pre-determine the nature of some of their findings.

For the essential problem the Sinclair Inquiry faced was a familiar one; namely, that the perpetrator of the killing was in contact with the appropriate authorities and that relevant information about him (and it is invariably a 'him') was known by some of those parties although either not shared, not properly understood, or not acted upon. The Report makes a series of recommendations about how to facilitate better communication, to ensure proper record taking, to supervise, train and support staff, to listen to families, and for all staff to have access to expert medical advice, especially in forensic issues. The impression that the Report leaves is that things could have been done better, more detailed systems should be in place and that individuals erred, even if not culpably so. Thus, 'All of this demonstrates a fragmentary style of care planning and operation, totally inadequate to meet the needs of a chronically ill patient. We conclude that the process was unstructured, unreviewed, uncommunicative and unsafe' (Lingham *et al.* 1996: para 5.4.6). However, is this finding of 'poor communication' inevitable? This is not to suggest that mental health services and social work departments are staffed with people who are in some way less competent or less caring than they ought to be, although it is self-evident that inter- and intra-agency communication are only as good as the people who do the communicating and that good communication takes time. Rather, it is to suggest that 'to err is human'. Inquiries into plane crashes – despite extensive training, regular medical assessments of staff and 'high-tech' equipment with fail-safe mechanisms – regularly attribute accidents to 'pilot error'. Or, as Reason (cited in Tidmarsh 1997) puts it:

All human beings, regardless of their skills, abilities and specialist knowledge, make fallible decisions and commit unsafe acts. This human propensity for committing errors and violating safety procedures can be moderated by selection, training, well-designed equipment and good management, but it can never be entirely eliminated.

Undoubtedly, a thorough investigation will always reveal inadequacies in a human service. As services managing those with mental disorder involve a high human input, they are particularly vulnerable. First, one does not need to be an organisations expert to recognise that people have lives away from their jobs, which can impact on them negatively, requiring them to take leave unexpectedly. Temporary cover may be provided, or the burden may be taken up by others, or matters sometimes just left in abeyance. Although disaster rarely follows (confirming the view that it is acceptable just to 'get by'), it is not unusual when disaster occurs for it to have been preceded by just such a period of personal stress amongst key workers. Second, as caring agencies, mental health and social services suffer from the additional disadvantage of having at the bottom end relatively poorly paid staff who have to learn much on the job, partly through extensive face-to-face contact with patients; they also experience the stress of coal-face caseloads. And of course, it is these people to whom patients may turn to make disclosures – as was the case in the Jason Mitchell Inquiry (see Peay 1997; Blom-Cooper *et al.* 1996). Yet such staff may lack confidence either in respect of the significance of what is being said, or what they should do with it, or because of concerns that their attempts to inform their seniors might rebound on them. At the top end of the structure, all of the stress that goes with consultant responsibility together with the requisite knowledge and experience of risk management, may interact with less frequent patient contact, so that consultants may obtain their information selectively, second-hand, in a corrupted form, or not at all.

Reasoning processes and responsibility

Here is not the place for a review of the now substantial literature on the psychology of decision-making. However, two features of that literature have particular relevance. First, the phenomenological complexity of legal decision-making does not necessarily reflect how decisions are actually made; simple decision strategies appear to be the rule rather than the exception (Hawkins 1986). Moreover, decision-making is not a model of calculated rationality; most importantly, it has a reflexive quality, being both anticipatory and backward looking. Second, we are all subject to limitations on our cognitive and processing abilities; two of these cognitive errors have particularly relevance; 'the fundamental attribution error' and the 'knew it all along effect' (Fitzmaurice and Pease 1986; Baron 1994). These are likely to impact on the inquiries' analyses: the fundamental attribution error arises because decision-makers are more likely to underestimate the influence of situational factors and overestimate dispositional factors in controlling behaviour. In crude terms, this leads them 'to attribute ineptitude to personal deficiencies rather than ignorance of situations' (Fitzmaurice and Pease 1986: 18). To illustrate, it is all too easy to attribute greater wisdom to Jeremy Paxman than the contestants on *University Challenge* because he has the opportunity to display his knowledge, and they their ignorance! For inquiries, the fundamental attribution error is most likely to contribute to the allocation of responsibility to individuals, at the expense of the explanatory force of the resource context in which they find themselves. The 'knew it all along effect' serves to exaggerate with hindsight what individuals could have been predicted to have known with foresight (hence, making them appear more 'blameworthy' for their errors). Specifically, hindsight tends to produce inflated perceptions of foreseeability and of the relevance of data preceding an event. If you ask people to predict the outcome of an event they will rate it much less likely than if they are told it has occurred. Which of us, for example, would have predicted that: (a) either of a pair of linked skydivers would have survived a parachute failure, or (b) that it was the novice who would have survived from a combination of novice and experienced skydiver? But knowing that this has occurred somehow makes the event seem more probable; this in turn not only leaves us with a sense that we understand the world, but also makes it peculiarly difficult for us to learn from events which ought to surprise us.

Taken together, as Fitzmaurice and Pease point out, the 'knew it all along effect' and the fundamental attribution error are likely to result in the concept of the reasonable man being systematically unfair to a defendant, since 'what is knowable to a reasonable man will be overstated, as will the independence of the reasonable man from situational pressures'(Fitzmaurice and Pease 1986: 32–33). As discussed below, this may have unwelcome consequences for assessments of negligence.

Although the inquiry reports may stress in their legally restrained conclusions that an event was neither predictable nor preventable, the devil is in the detail. The detail focuses on particular decisions and on pieces of information which were known or could have been known and asks, what if all of this had been put together? But the question remains whether, even if this information had been put together, would people's interpretations of it prospectively have matched the conclusions they reached retrospectively? Moreover, whilst the reports do not intend to condemn, they do criticise, and make observations on the actions and omissions of named staff without ever being able to reconstruct their behaviour in its context (of the time, stress, pressure, and other information possessed – ultimately irrelevant or redundant to the death – but pertinent at the time to that individual). There is also a tendency to highlight particular incidents as critical. Yet such incidents will also have occurred in a context, not just of a failure to act or to act too late by one party, but in the context of the acts and assumptions of others. Thus, it was not just that Ms Till didn't phone Dr Mikhail, but that he did not contact her either; and when she spoke to Ms Chater, between them they did nothing immediately. Inquiry reports rarely seek to establish what else the participants were doing at these critical moments, about what other disasters they may have unknowingly been averting. Whether, for example, Dr Mikhail's inaction in respect of Mr Sinclair was to the benefit of the relatives of Mr X, when Patient Y does not go on to kill? Finally, at inquiries any failure fully to record a past incident or play down a piece of criminal behaviour such as, for example, the downgrading of the attempted murder charge in the Jason Mitchell case (Blom-Cooper et al. 1996) or Andrew Robinson's assault on a previous girlfriend (Blom Cooper et al. 1995), can be highlighted as a significant error. Yet would this knowledge have made a difference to how someone was treated, or does it merely constitute 'part of the history'?[11] With all of these questions, it is regrettably impossible to examine the past without the knowledge of the homicide(s) influencing how the past is reconstructed and then weighed.

One further difficulty is also attributable to a common error of cognition; that is, that the availability of constructed reasons will increase the perceived probability of an outcome. Yet this is just what the inquiry process achieves; by chronologically charting the course of an event in an attempt to provide some understanding (and to learn some lessons) of what happened, they provide potentially spurious grounds for an assessment that the event was more probable than it was. Eastman describes this as the 'risk of inferring culpability by dint of describing causal responsibility' (1996: 1070), but one could go even further. Does an inevitably partial and selective description of what happened seduce us into a form of reasoning which implies with hindsight that there are things we *should* have foreseen, because they appear more probable than they actually were once we have described the process which preceded them? Does the inquiry process therefore stop at the point at which an explanation (which makes the events seem probable) emerges, without going further or deeper to look for additional, competing or conflicting explanations? In connection with this, Carson explores the contrasting approaches of inquiries and courts, noting for example, the requirement that courts be satisfied according to a designated threshold (whether it be beyond reasonable doubt, on a balance of probabilities, etc.), whereas we have no means of knowing, when inquiries draw conclusions, what confidence they have in them, and therefore what significance we should attach to them (Carson 1996).

Clunis: wrecked or scuttled?

The Court of Appeal struck out Christopher Clunis' action against Camden and Islington Health Authority as revealing no cause of action arising from failure by the defendant health authority or Dr Seargeant to carry out their functions under s.117 of the Mental Health Act 1983. Moreover, the court did not think it would be fair or reasonable to hold the defendant responsible for the consequences of Clunis' criminal act.[12] Clunis had contended that he had suffered injury, loss and damage because the health authority were negligent and were responsible for a breach of duty of care at common law to treat him with reasonable professional care and skill. Dr Seargeant, in particular, was alleged to have been negligent in the way in which she carried out her responsibilities 'for monitoring the implementation of the patient's care plan and liaising and co-ordinating where necessary between the individuals and agencies involved in it'. Although the Court of Appeal's judgement refers to Dr Seargeant as 'a key worker' (transcript p.6), the Inquiry Report is somewhat more trenchant:

> Dr Seargeant left too much to the Social Services Department when she should have been taking an active role. She did not involve her Consultant, Dr Taylor, in managing this difficult case. As the person *named as keyworker* under the S117 Mental Health Act 1983 aftercare plan, Dr Seargeant knew that if she did not do so, no one else would.
>
> (Ritchie *et al*. 1994: 88, emphasis added)

And later in the Report, after commenting favourably on the actions of Ursula Robson, an approved social worker employed by Haringey Social Services, who had 'in the space of a few hours [done] more to find out about Christopher Clunis than others had done over the previous two months', the Report notes: 'She was delayed by the continuing uncertainty from Dr Seargeant as to which psychiatric service would be responsible for Christopher Clunis' (ibid.: para 38.2.1).

Dr Seargeant was not, of course, the only professional criticised by the Report for indecision and procrastination; for example, the Report found Inspector Gill

> knew that it was Christopher Clunis who had been waving a screwdriver in the streets and talking about devils... He should have realised that Christopher Clunis was a danger to the public and probably to himself . . . he did nothing to ensure that Christopher Clunis was safe. It is our view that the police were thereby not properly protecting the public from potential harm.
>
> (ibid.: para 36.2.3)

Yet the Court of Appeal seemingly used the position of the police to bolster their argument about why the statutory framework of the Mental Health Act did not create a duty to take care, breach of which can give rise to a claim for damages.[13] However, the thinking revealed seems less than rigorous, since the court has juxtaposed the difficulty of holding Dr Seargeant responsible alongside similar failures by the police. Are the two directly comparable, though? The Report is critical of the police, but it does not appear that the police were ever in a position on any occasion to exercise their s.136 powers; accordingly, failure to do so may be less than negligent, even though the criticism could be made that the police might have made more effort to put themselves into a position where Clunis could have been apprehended before the homicide occurred. In contrast, Dr Seargeant's specific responsibilities under s.117 were continuing; failure to fulfil her duties as named keyworker were coterminous. In short, just because responsibilities for the mentally disordered are diffused, this should not imply that no one is responsible.

Even if the Court of Appeal are correct in their interpretation of the statutory framework, their rejection of the submission that a parallel duty of care in common law exists for discharged patients is curious. The judgement observes these duties of care to be 'different in nature from those owed by a doctor to a patient whom he is treating' (and for breach of which the authority would be liable). However, can this be right in an era when the bulk of care is non-hospital based? Or is the Court drawing a spurious distinction on the basis that, although named as keyworker, Dr Seargeant had not actually carried out her first assessment? If so, this would seem to encourage delay in the provision of services, rather than to facilitate them, as s.117 was specifically intended so to do.

Of course, had the action not been struck out then the court would have had to have been satisfied on a balance of probabilities that the practitioners fell short of a standard of care that would be employed by at least some responsible body of their own profession holding that post.[14] The question then arises – might this standard of care be vulnerable to 'enhancement' were there to be widespread dissemination of the inquiry's assorted recommendations? Although some enhancement might well be desirable, is there a risk that an enhanced standard might be set inappropriately high, because of the cognitive errors to which the inquiries are necessarily subject?

A glimmer of an answer is evident from the litigation following *The Herald of Free Enterprise* disaster.[15] Lay people might argue that it is self-evidently negligent for a cross-Channel ferry to leave port with its bow doors open. But if all ferry operators did this, and no mishap occurs, is it negligent? Or have they all just been lucky? Gobert refers to this as the 'fortuity of consequence' and argues that just because one has been lucky, does not make one not negligent (Gobert 1994: 724). However, once an accident has occurred, it shifts the perception of risk and presumably therefore, the retrospective assessment as to whether one was prospectively negligent. Although the question of whether an 'obvious and serious risk' was created when the *Herald* set forth with her bow doors open was never resolved, the Judge, the Sheen Inquiry, and the Law Commission were all seemingly prepared to infer that if other companies had precautions in place, this might create a legitimate basis for such a deduction. This would seem to imply that the more reports published detailing ways in which mental health professionals can err, the greater is the likelihood if they don't adapt their practices (while others do), they will be found negligent. Even if a practitioner could point to similarly placed professionals who had not adapted their practices, would they be regarded by either the courts or the profession as a 'responsible body' or as 'reasonably competent'?

However, this may be a bear trap with significant implications for patient care. In an ideal world, the inquiries' recommendations would serve to raise standards generally, improving patient care and creating a higher threshold against which to provide redress where professionals fall short. But in the real world another consequence may ensue. To produce good practice you need guidelines. The more guidelines you have, the greater is the possibility that you will fall short of them. Thus, Monahan (thinking with his liability hat on) has argued that it may be better to have no policy than to have one that you do not fully implement (1993). Down this route lies defensive medicine, but a form of defensive medicine that means doing not more unnecessary tests, but asking fewer necessary questions. Thus, some practitioners may refrain from asking some questions for fear of being fixed with the knowledge that an answer may bring, preferring instead to rely upon the 'fortuity of consequence'.

One other consequence may result from the climate of litigiousness. The detail of the inquiry reports reveal that no matter how many good practice guidelines get produced, the effectiveness of their implementation depends upon matters more ephemeral than the mere rigour with which they are circulated. For it is the quality of relationships between staff and the confidence that they have in one another that will encourage them to share their own anxieties about patients. It is hard to imagine a guideline which says 'Do not hold back for fear of looking silly', but easy to think of properly resourced supervisory relationships which would encourage this. But they are unlikely to be created or sustained where staff spend their time looking over their shoulders.

Concluding this chapter is not easy, for the arguments will be ongoing. It is to be hoped that *Clunis* does not ultimately block the path of litigation; equally, it is to be hoped that the inquiry industry will recognise that as much as is likely to be learnt has been laid bare, while some of its lessons are best relegated as a reflection of the inevitability of human error, rather than as a testament to human wickedness.

Acknowledgements

The themes in this chapter were aired first at a seminar organised by St George's Hospital Medical School in July 1997. I am grateful for the comments I received then.

Notes

1 Homicides are rare events; those by psychiatric patients rarer still; and those by psychiatric patients of strangers so rare as to be remarkable. Indeed, the latest published findings indicate that of 408 homicide convictions in the study, only 12 per cent were perpetrated by those who had had contact with the mental health services during the 12 months before their offences. Moreover, when the mentally disordered killed, they were most likely to kill their own family members; strangers constituted only 10 per cent of their victims (for the mentally well, 'strangers' constituted 26 per cent of their victims) Appleby Report, *The Guardian*, 12 December 1997 broadly replicating the findings of Sims A. (Chair) (1996) *Report of the Confidential Inquiry into Homicides and Suicides by Mentally Ill People*, Royal College of Psychiatrists. Copies available from 17 Belgrave Square, London SW1X 8PG). The Appleby Report explodes (again) one other common misconception about the mentally ill, by clearly demonstrating that they are more dangerous to themselves than others; killings by those who have had contact with the psychiatric services occur on average once per week, but some 20 people a week in this group commit suicide.

2 This, of course, is in addition to the blame they probably anyway heap upon themselves It is a common cognitive error to overestimate one's own centrality to events and underestimate the centrality of others. Such error leads victims of crime and other disasters to blame themselves; health care professionals are unlikely to be immune to such processes.

3 *Christopher Clunis (by his next friend Christopher Prince) v Camden and Islington Health Authority*. CA. Judgement given 5 December 1997. QBENI 97/0044/E. In fact, the judgement turns upon whether any such duty exists, rather than the standard of care required before the duty might be breached. Whilst the Clunis case will be argued by some to have a relatively narrow impact, it is important to note that the decision is likely to ripple across the landscape of out-of-court settlements. It is likely to contribute to a much more robust attitude by Health and/or Local Authorities when these tragedies occur.

4 These two overriding themes have been succinctly put as 'not every tragedy can be prevented [but] every service can be improved' in one of the latest inquiry reports; Lingham R and Candy J. (1997) *Inquiry into the Treatment and Care of Damian*

Witts. Summary of the Report commissioned by Gloucestershire Health Authority. December 1997 at p. 29.

5 See for example *Monitor, The Journal of the Zito Trust* 1997 Issue no. 2 which classifies a large number of homicides by former psychiatric patients as being 'stranger' killings This is due partly to an analysis which has adopted a broad definition of stranger; for example, the killing of Brian Bennett by Stephen Laudat, both of whom attended the same day care centre, comes within this ambit.

6 Although suing the perpetrator is the legally obvious solution, perpetrators are unlikely to have any resources, unless they have been able successfully to sue the relevant health authority for its breaches; in this context, Jayne Zito supported Clunis' action against the health authority.

7 See the oft cited *Holgate and Another v Lancashire Mental Hospital Board, Gill and Robertson* [1937] 4 KBD 19.

8 The case of *Meah v McCreamer (No. 1)* [1985] 1 All ER 367. Much beloved by teachers of tort law, the plaintiff recovered damages based on his conviction for two rapes which took place after he suffered a head injury in a road accident. The Court of Appeal did not regard this as authoritative, as the issue of public policy (i.e. whether a wrongdoing plaintiff can recover damages) had not been raised explicitly.

9 My title is, in fact, a corruption of an early edition of *ER* in which young Dr Carter spends the entire episode exploring rare diagnoses with an elderly patient only ultimately to discover that she is suffering from Alzheimer's disease.

10 An exploratory discussion of these issues took place at the Royal College of Psychiatrists Special Interest Group in Philosophy meeting in Southampton, Feb–March 1997 – J. Peay (1996) 'The responsible psychiatrist: doctoring autonomy'.

11 In the criminal process, the rules of evidence would regulate the use of such prejudicial information; yet, at inquiries their significance is arguably overplayed and unrestrained.

12 Leave to appeal to the House of Lords was refused.

13 As the Court of Appeal noted, s.136 empowers a constable finding a mentally disordered person to be in immediate need of care and control to remove that person to a place of safety. The Court doubted whether even the specificity of this language would create the relevant duty to take care.

14 *Bolam v Frien Hospital Management Committee* [1957] 2 All ER 118.

15 Although it is normally dangerous to draw parallels between criminal and civil cases, negligence in corporate manslaughter requires a gross breach of the requisite standard, making it arguably more robust than the civil test.

References

Baron, J. (1994) *Thinking and Deciding*. Cambridge: Cambridge University Press

Blom-Cooper, L., Grounds, A., Guinan, P., Parker, A. and Taylor, M. (1996) *The Case of Jason Mitchell: Report of the Independent Panel of Inquiry*. London: Duckworth.

Blom-Cooper, L., Hally, H. and Murphy, E. (1995) *The Falling Shadow: One Patient's Mental Health Care, 1978–1993*. London: Duckworth.

Carson D. (1996) 'Structural problems, perspectives and solutions'. In J. Peay (ed.) *Inquiries after Homicide*. London: Duckworth.

Crichton, J. and Sheppard, D. (1996) 'Psychiatric inquiries: learning the lessons'. In J. Peay (ed.) *Inquiries after Homicide*. London: Duckworth.

Department of Health (1994) *Guidance on the Discharge of Mentally Disordered People and their Continuing Care in the Community*. London: NHS Executive HSG(94)27.

—— (1995) *Building Bridges. A Guide to Arrangements for Inter-Agency Working for the Care and Protection of Severely Mentally Ill People*. London: HMSO.

Eastman, N. (1996) 'Inquiry into homicides by psychiatric patients: systematic audit should replace mandatory inquiries'. *British Medical Journal* 313, 1069–1071.

Fitzmaurice, C. and Pease, K. (1986) *The Psychology of Judicial Sentencing*. Manchester: Manchester University Press.

Gobert, J. (1994) 'Corporate criminality: new crimes for the times'. *Criminal Law Review* 722–734.

Hawkins, K. (1986) 'On legal decision-making'. *Washington and Lee Law Review* 43 (4), 1161–1242.

Lingham, R., Candy, J. and Bray, J. (1996) *The Report of the Inquiry into the Treatment and Care of Raymond Sinclair*. West Kent Health Authority and Kent County Council Social Services.

Monahan, J. (1993) 'Limiting therapist exposure to *Tarasoff* liability. Guidelines for risk containment'. *American Psychologist* 48 (3), 242–250.

—— (1996) 'The MacArthur violence risk assessment study: An executive summary of the research of the working group'. Proceedings of the MacArthur Foundation Research Network *Violence, Competence and Coercion: The Pivotal Issues in Mental Health Law*. Wadham College, Oxford 3–4 July.

Peay J. (ed.) (1996) *Inquiries after Homicide*. London: Duckworth.

—— (1997) 'Clinicians and inquiries: demons, drones or demigods?' *International Review of Psychiatry* 9 (2–3), 171–177.

Petch, E. and Bradley, C. (1997) 'Learning the lessons from homicide inquiries: adding insult to injury?' *Journal of Forensic Psychiatry* 8 (2), 161–184.

Prins, H. (1996) 'Risk assessment and management in criminal justice and psychiatry'. *Journal of Forensic Psychiatry* 7 (1), 42–62.

Reder, P. and Duncan, S. (1996) 'Reflections on child abuse inquiries'. In J. Peay (ed.) *Inquiries after Homicide*. London: Duckworth.

Reder, P., Duncan, S. and Gray, M. (1993) *Beyond Blame: Child Abuse Tragedies Revisited*. London: Routledge.

Reiner R. (1998) 'Copping a plea'. In S. Holdaway and P. Rock (eds) *The Social Theory of Criminology*. London: UCL Press.

Ritchie, J. (Chairman), Dick, D. and Lingham, R. (1994) *The Report of the Inquiry into the Care and Treatment of Christopher Clunis*. London: HMSO.

Shepphard, D. (1996) *Learning the Lessons: Mental Health Inquiry Reports Published in England and Wales 1969–1996 and their Recommendations for Improving Practice*. 2nd edn. London: Zito Trust.

Tidmarsh, D. (1997) 'Psychiatric risk, safety cultures and homicide inquiries'. *Journal of Forensic Psychiatry* 8 (2), 138–151.

Chapter 10

A balance of possibilities

Some concluding notes on rights, risks and the mentally disordered offender

David Webb

There is no one body of knowledge that holds a monopoly either of concern for, or explanatory authority towards, the mentally disordered offender. Contributors to this book have reflected that plurality, with elements drawn from both the administrative and the critical domains of criminology, from the interventive narratives of probation practice and social work, and from socio-legal perspectives on the 'processing' of those who are both mentally ill and are offenders.

This book began with a chapter written by an outsider, who, while familiar with the broad disciplines that bear in on the subject of the mentally disordered offender, professed no immediate familiarity with the substantive matter at hand. The same goes for this concluding piece, where some form of sociology guides how matters are to be approached. There is a definite connection, though, between the interests of the specialist and those of the academic outsider. Society's reaction to the complex amalgam made up of an individual status on which is inscribed both mental disorder, and a delinquency of conduct that announces criminality, says much about the wider culture of which the phenomenon is a part, and it is this which offers the entrée for the generalist. Returning to the broad sweep, this concluding chapter draws on – and, we hope, draws out – some of the themes offered by our specialist contributors. Above all it focuses on one of the particularly enduring narratives within what is written on this subject, namely that we continue to find this fragment of human waywardness (requiring as it does an unstable mixture of care, control, punishment, medication, tolerance, watchfulness), so repeatedly perplexing that there remains the suspicion that the amount of talk is in inverse proportion to the securing of anything even remotely approaching a solution. Matters have not been helped by the fact that the area has become so ideologically contested, so wracked by debates that reach to the heart of contemporary western thinking that it is difficult sometimes to see a way out of these various positions. Higgins (somewhat despairingly) characterises the disputed territory that is occupied by our consideration of the mentally disordered offender as

> the disturbance of the settled, cosy and pragmatic relationship between
> psychiatrists, courts and the bureaucracy by the appearance of civil liberties

lawyers and criminologists raising issues such as: the right to be punished; the right not to be punished; the right to be treated; the right not to be treated; the justice of indeterminate sentences especially when associated with treatments of debatable efficacy; and the poor predictability of dangerousness.

(Higgins 1984: 11)

With all this stacked up against the topic of managing the mentally disordered offender, it is perhaps surprising that any headway at all is made in moving constructively forward. Of course we hope that our contributors have indeed effected some progress on these matters, in line with the hammering out of advances in this perplexing field that has characterised the interventions made by Herschel Prins himself over the years.

Despite the occasionally labyrinthine disquisitions on the subject of the mentally disordered offender, the topic has sometimes seemed deceptively straightforward, and we can do no better than be reminded once again of matters with an economical statement from Seymour Halleck:

> Mentally disordered offenders are formally identified on the basis of two general criteria. First, the evidence that they have committed a crime must be sufficient to lead to their arrest and arraingement. Second, an agency of the criminal justice system must suspect that they have a mental disorder of such proportion as to question the fairness and utility of subjecting them to the usual criminal justice process.
>
> (Halleck 1987:1)

The consequential *principles* of intervention are themselves more or less straightforward – again on the face of it. The administration of justice demands both equity and fairness – that concern for what Hudson notes as 'individuality, singularity, the precise match of remedy to situation' (1996: 156). This is so that there should be some form of relationship which is self-evident, and widely supported, between a particular infraction of the legal code and what society subsequently sanctions by way of the penalty that must be borne by the wrongdoer. This of course, rests on the assumption that all individuals have the capacity to understand that their actions will indeed lead to certain outcomes, and that they grasp that they might at some future moment be held to account for the rightness or wrongness of their actions. But in so far as there are in fact differing capacities to control behaviour, so it follows – at least in the kinds of humane jurisdictions that Herschel Prins enjoins us to adhere to – that there should be differential treatment of that behaviour. As Halleck again rather nicely expresses it, 'the quest for fairness and beneficence limits the severity of retribution based on the notion of desert' (1987: 19).

These are matters addressed through what might be called 'substantive justice'. This is less to do with the formal application of invariant rules, but rather a concern with the way in which those rules might be given appropriate interpretation in specific instances. The resulting attention to the particularities of this or that individual case, while demanding flexibility, discretion and interpretation, means that the longer-term legitimacy of those rules is that much more secure. In his chapter Robert Harris talks about the way in which this is resolved in Britain through the blending of formal statute with common law, so that while sentencing 'by the book' generally occurs, it need not do so, if good sense suggests that the characteristics of the offender demand otherwise. Due consideration of individual circumstances can thereby be introduced flexibly, and without disruption to the overall 'framework' of law. Those with demonstrably lower or lesser levels of competence, blameworthiness and responsibility thereby become exempt from the strict application of formal rules governing the administration of punishment. This, though, puts something of a functionalist gloss on the pragmatics of jurisprudence: the way in which the medico-juridical 'system' operates towards mentally disordered offenders might indeed create the *impression* of humanity for those wrong-doers who are without reason. In his contribution, John Wood suggests that a certain symbolism of attentiveness in reviewing the incarceration of the mentally ill (through the machinery of the Mental Health Review Tribunals) is the thing that matters, almost irrespective of the infrequency of successful appeal. Likewise, Judith Pitchers' discussion of the operation of parole applications for mentally disordered offenders paints a picture which could be construed as a process driven more by the caution of professional and institutional interests than by the application of reasonably well-informed risk assessments. In short, the whole business of managing the mentally disordered offender is shot through with equivocation and hesitancy. It is for this reason that as a sub-title for this book we have taken – or rather adapted slightly – a telling phrase from one of Herschel Prins's papers: 'the people nobody owns' (Prins 1994), since this conveys if not the statelessness of these citizens, then their 'statuslessness' – internal refugees moving between administrative domains which only accept them with reluctance and on a temporary basis.

A test of the civilising process[1]

The mentally disordered offender presents a series of 'tests' to challenge the capacity of society to respond to its wayward citizens who are not only troubled in themselves, but who are also troublesome to others (Craft 1984; Shah 1993). Their disturbed psychological state sets them firmly within the social deviancy of mental illness, and in transgressing the moral boundary between observing the law and breaking it, they are also demonstrably 'criminal'. In this way the mentally disordered offender has been subject to two particularly significant and powerful social censures – mental illness as the judgement over rightness of mind, and the imputation of deviance as a judgement about behavioural admission to civilised society, though in truth they are treated more on the basis of the former, (the status of what he or she *is*) than on the basis of their conduct (what he or she has *done*) (Duff and Garland 1995). We do not need much reminding that society is especially fearful of offenders who doubly transgress: those who are not only law breakers, but who in their mental deviancy are outside the domains of rational cognition, carefully modulated affect and the sophisticated role-playing that are demanded by the complexities of modern times.

These are people whose 'role performance' is severally compromised, and in their waywardness they fall under the tutelage of two of modern society's most powerful professions – medicine and the law. The claim of these occupational groups to speak authoritatively on the subject is sometimes competitive: presuming the rationality of human agency and of the willed nature of wrong-doing, legal concerns have had to acknowledge that incapacitated mental processes constrain the applicability – as well as the legitimacy – of what might be called 'pure' legalism (Busfield 1996). But if the law has been held in check when it comes to the formal enforcement of retributive justice, this is not to say that there has been wholesale and successful diversion from the criminal justice system to more appropriate domains of social intervention. Far from it. More often than not, these people are caught between hospital and prison. Consequences of the reluctance (or at best the conditional willingness) to set the treatment of mentally disordered offenders within the domain of mental health, despite a long-standing policy commitment to doing just this, is a recurrent theme in Herschel Prins's work, and is echoed here in this collection. What are ostensibly rights granted to mentally disordered offenders under statute, such that they might be entitled to appropriate health care to meet their illness, become instead further limitations on their freedom if the machinery to implement that protection is either ill-designed or poorly maintained. Not surprisingly, there is a view – widely and respectably held – that those who are mentally disordered are too frequently managed within the criminal justice system, for no other reason that the capacity of psychiatric provision – whether institutional or community-based – is simply unable, or unwilling to add another risk to those that it would be carrying anyway. In so far as recourse to criminal justice reflects the inadequacy of mental health care, then there must be serious concerns about the rights of people who ought to be 'patients'. As Judith Pitchers argues in the conclusion of her chapter, the tendency to play safe so far as mentally disordered offenders are concerned – the case with which she is concerned being that of parole – does indeed lead to injustices for particular individuals being accepted as unfortunate, if inevitable, expressions of that most enduring utilitarian maxim – the greatest good of the greatest number.

Halleck refers to the alternating tendency to meddle and to ignore that marks the social reaction to people whose existence confronts our sometimes flawed capacity to address the philosophical complexities around mind, disorder and crime. 'We are unwilling to leave them alone', he writes, 'yet most agencies seek to avoid responsibility for their care. We confine them to prisons and to prison-like hospitals where they are sometimes treated worse than offenders' (Halleck 1987: 11).

Various professional domains ostensibly responsible for mentally disordered offenders do not always sit easily together, and again the literature is replete with the complexities arising from the almost ineluctable imperative of multi-professional collaboration when faced with people whose problems are impossible to set with any one disciplinary or professional discourse (see Preston-Shoot; Grant, this volume). Against this particular logic which points to working together, is another that leads in the opposite direction. The empirical and common-sensical underpinnings of the law, easily connecting with taken-for-granted everyday ideas about wrong-doing, have to reach an accommodation with something altogether more difficult and arcane. The business of assessing mental processes, while relying almost invariably on the observable behaviour of the individual, is often suspected of deriving from something that is part witchcraft, part mumbo-jumbo. And of course, there is always the deeply held suspicion that anyone who would seek to account for the impact of mental incapacity on wrong-doing is simply trading in excuse-mongering, something which occasionally sees itself being played out in the very public gaze of celebrated criminal trials. So it was in the case of Peter Sutcliffe that the unseemly disputes between rival psychiatrists did nothing for the jury, who rejected entirely any idea that the defendant was mentally disturbed, but was instead simply culpable for his horrific actions. (See Prins 1983).

Fathoming out the respective weights of madness and badness when explaining wayward behaviour is exemplified when thinking about 'criminals' who are also mentally ill. We might recognise that these people are incapable of meeting the tests of rationality, culpability and capability that underpin admission to judicial processing and sanction, and indeed the diverting of them from the criminal justice system is regarded – as it is by Paul Cavadino in this volume – as essential if we are to operate a humane approach to those offenders whose reasons for law-breaking are unintelligible. But as the case of Sutcliffe reminds us, there is always the residual cultural sentiment that sees offenders who are mentally disordered as somehow escaping the criminal sanction if they receive medical treatment that smacks of 'therapy' (Hodgins, 1993). Sometimes this still shapes the social reaction to offenders who are mentally disordered, towards whom the residual cultural predilections of Benthamite justice-grinding are directed (Peay, 1994). Seemingly, neither professionals, nor state agencies are exempt from this fixation with the almost exclusively corporeal, with for example McConville (1995: 284) pointing out that '(p)rison medical services, obsessed with malingering, have always been more at ease with bodily rather than mental illness'. The fact that so often mentally ill people (whose condition, even without the assessment of an 'expert' would point them towards being self-evidently 'patients') find them-selves in prison, suggests that whether by occasional lapses into prejudice by those who are involved in the everyday workings of juridical–welfare adminis-tration, or because of the kinds of 'structural' failings in the system that are described for example by Philip Bean in this book, we have yet to resolve certain of these ambiguities in the management of this particular social deviance.

Actuarial welfare and managing the mentally disordered offender

The history of the way in which mentally disordered people have been 'managed' is replete with the outrages that have been visited upon them – sometimes out of fear, sometimes out of ignorance and sometimes out of a misplaced sense of doing good (see for example, Donnelly 1983; Sedgewick 1982). Added to this is the ease with which battalions of critics have been able to 'deconstruct' the very existence of mental disorder, showing it to be the consequence of social labelling, or arising from the iniquities of particular societies and their failings in, say, distributive justice. Not surprisingly, this legacy of anti-psychiatry and labelling theory rings hollow to those for whom mental illness has a powerful, limiting and materially constraining reality to it (Sedgewick 1982). And in cultures under the sway of rationalist, individualistic ways of thinking, mental disorder – with its connotations of behaviour driven not so much by human agency but by some sort of motivational corruption arising from an ill mind – has to compete with an inclination to regard human action as intended and as consequentially aware.

The determination of mental illness more often than not entails a measure of judgement by the person making the assessment, and it is because of this that the various categories of mental disorder have been sometimes seen as being 'socially constructed'. By this is meant that diagnoses are less the reflection of secure scientific knowledge, and more the product of moral evaluations about various forms of socially unacceptable behaviour that vary and alter across time and space. There is also a view that the determination of what stands as 'dangerous' is indeed dependent on certain mores, with particular groups more likely than others to fall within this estimation of potential disruption. In his chapter Paul Cavadino suggests that it is precisely this that applies to black offenders, echoing a point that was made in the report into the death of Orville Blackwood chaired by Herschel Prins (Prins, 1993c). The assumptions and 'typifications' that are held about black people by those with front-line responsibilities for containment and care in the prison hospital have self-fulfilling consequences, not only for those who are being treated or contained (who may 'take on' the attributions to which they are subject through social labelling), but also for those charged with their supervision.

These few observations – let alone those that have accumulated in the preceding pages – serve as a reminder that to speak of 'managing' members of this social group is to invite a measure of controversy. Might not there be something impersonally 'technical' about this subject? To talk of 'management' perhaps shows that we are not really concerned with the *care* of our fellow citizens who have a disturbance in their mental functioning. Rather, we want to 'take charge' of them, and subject them to the surveillance and regulation to which we habitually subject the various deviants who disturb conventions of the moral order. Or does the reference to management echo the medical discourse within which troubles of the mind have to be coaxed or driven to submission, in the same way that physical illness or disease is brought under control? 'Management' – the casually dismissive may say – regards those who are mentally ill as objects to whom things are done. But there is an alternative interpretation, one which we believe reflects something of the approach taken by Herschel Prins (see Prins 1994).

Management implies the coordination of resources and service provision and the shaping of policy in order to meet desired objectives, and much of this book has referred to how this might be done. It need not necessarily refer to direct involvement with individual offenders, but with a wider reach of concerns. Webster and Menzies convey with some feeling this idea of management as having 'system-wide' properties when they set down proposals to address the deficiencies in services for mentally disordered offenders that they identified in their study of a large North American city:

> The challenge must be one of sitting with administrators and planners from various government ministries, including housing authorities, in the hope that we can create a 'hybrid' scheme that will reduce the imposition of actually unnecessary sentences, lower criminal recidivism and at the same time improve the mental, physical and social well-being of such unfortunate people so evidently in need.
>
> (Webster and Menzies 1993: 36)

The term 'management' conveys, not entirely inappropriately, the ascendency of the actuarial over earlier narratives that spoke of individualised medical or welfare 'treatment'. This line of arguing maintains that rather than the reformist goal of what Pearson (1975) refers to as the restoration of the deviant to 'utility' (so that they might come to share in the values of the community), the new actuarial regime looks to the careful calculation of risk and the efficient deployment of resources at those for whom predictive indications suggest that they pose the greatest threat (Hudson 1996: 154). The goal of welfare actuarialism is to warn in advance of human behaviour taking place – to engage in the corporate manager's equivalent of 'future proofing' by anticipating the consequences that will flow from a careful uncovering of the 'signs' that are all around us, yet to which so many are oblivious. The 'reading' of an individual's biography in order to reveal their code of abnormality, and the assigning of this to a particular category within a taxonomy of ideal-typical waywardness, is a way of generating security of knowledge in a world that otherwise would be marked by randomly bizarre behaviour.

As it happens, an insistence on fact garnering for the purposes of prediction had earlier seen its place in Prins's recommendations to practitioners (Prins 1975), though the writer of the present chapter took some exception to this, arguing that we only tend to know why facts are pertinent once we re-construct preceding salience with the benefit of retrospective interpretation (Webb 1976). It is something that Jill Peay refers to in her contribution as the exaggeration with hindsight of what we could have predicted with foresight. In fact, if we were to identify not so much thematic continuity in Herschel Prins's work as a gentle realignment, it would point to a movement from the pursuit of positivist certitude about individual psychological malfunctioning, to a probabilistic and contingency-slanted approach. In this, the interactions between individual offenders and the apparatus of the criminal justice system figure more prominently in 'creating' a symptomatology which is more to do with what Busfield (1996) calls the 'role performance' of the mentally disordered than with a reductionist psycho-physiology.

In any event, there seems to be a wide recognition that predictive diagnoses of dangerousness are often inaccurate, leading to obvious concerns about punishing, or 'treating' people not so much for something they have done, but for what they might do – or perhaps more importantly, what they might not do (Duff and Garland: 1995). This of course echoes what we have already said about the 'category confusion' that dogs almost everything about the mentally disordered offender – between, on the one hand, the status of who they are, and, on the other, the conduct in which they have engaged. The tendency – in the administration of risk taking – is to play safe, as several of our contributors have shown.

Nevertheless, it has to be acknowledged that incapacitating the potential wrong-doer might well protect the community, even if this limits the rights of individuals about whom we are merely suspicious rather than certain. This does depend, though, on minimising the errors of false positives such that the abrogation of contract between citizenry and state is not jeopardised without legitimate warrant. The careful balance demanded by this set of simultaneous imperatives makes the business of risk assessment that much more important. Morris argues that the most robust basis for predictive intervention, and what he calls 'risk shifting', is indeed the actuarial. In this, the evidence is assembled to show that people who are like the particular offender before us, situated within the same conditions as is 'our' offender, have behaved in a certain way in the past. Given the similarity between the individual and the generality, the inference can be drawn (with varying degrees of confidence) that the person in question will behave in the future as others in the same position behaved in the past (Morris 1995). Theoretically at least, this approach might point towards a mechanism for limiting the uncertainty in the management of the mentally disordered offender, such that some sort of equilibrium is reached between the right of the community to be protected, and the right of the individual not to be incapacitated without warrant.

It is something of a recurrent theme in this collection that there is a special significance when the mentally disordered person is also an offender, for this points to an accumulation of jeopardy in the face of social control which is invoked to meet the multi-dimensionality of moral transgression (see also Shah 1993). The fact of mental disorder and the unpredictabilities in conduct that arise from disturbances in mental functioning are indeed socially troublesome. However, recognising that society itself has a responsibility to those of its members who are rendered vulnerable through their own misfortunes may have some merit:

'a danger to themselves or to others' remains the basis for the socially sanctioned restraint of those who are mentally disordered, and within this it is possible to discern the germ of a principle that recognises, as Rotman (1995) argues, for rehabilitation as a constitutional right; a duty owed by the state to the imprisoned mentally ill. It is this paternalistic obligation which finds expression in the principle of *parens patriae*, where the state assumes to itself the care of those of its citizens who cannot care for themselves, offenders or not.

Central to such an obligation is the accountability which must follow in the wake of any failure in discharging that appropriated duty with proper care. It is this which presumably lies behind Louis Blom-Cooper's staunch advocacy of public rather than private hearings when things have gone wrong, since these represent a greater good to the community than the harm that might befall those who have to account for their actions within these open forums. Of course, the point at which responsibility rests when what Rotman calls 'a constitutional right' (or we might term 'natural justice') is abrogated is a moot point. When it comes to restoring the social contract between wronged citizens and those in whose charge they have been placed, both Blom-Cooper and Jill Peay touch on the difficulty of assigning culpability to individuals (through professional negligence, for example) as against an indictment of diffuse social arrangements, such as 'racist cultures' in Special Hospitals, though our sense is that increasingly – and rather encouragingly – adverse 'social arrangements' are seen to be somebody's responsibility, and often this is someone occupying a position of some power.

Embedded within the way in which we approach the management of the mentally disordered offender are those calculations concerned with the likely danger posed to the community by the disturbed law breaker. It is for precisely this reason that the detailed forensic understanding of these various disturbed states – and their likely behavioural *sequelae* – is of such importance. Once another utilitarian axiom, namely that of universal capability, is questioned, then the principle of automatic punishment for infractions can be that more easily set aside. If the mentally disordered offender is not judged to be dangerous either to themselves or to the community, then the objectives of management can be beneficent, whereas if dangerous, the case is made for specialised programmes which are principally concerned with social protection (see Halleck 1987).

However – and fine principle notwithstanding – it is perhaps not surprising that this area of work is sometimes marked by vacillation in both policy and in professional practice. It is more than an intellectual or cognitive matter. It is true that the co-presence of mind, disorder and crime – all of which are themselves of enormous substantive, philosophical and moral complexity – makes the mentally disordered offender an especially challenging category to think about (Hollin and Howells 1993). But beyond this is something less amenable to such a distancing narrative. Herschel Prins himself has pointed out that managing the mentally disordered offender poses many challenges, often of an existential nature, and that the subjective feelings of those working in this field need to be acknowledged. Coming to terms with revulsion at horrific or bizarre acts, or coping with disruptions in thought processes which are both profoundly irrational yet firmly held; reconciling the competing responsibilities towards the rights of the offender on the one hand and the interests of the public on the other; the high personal investment that is made once a particular therapeutic path is taken to address complex difficulties – all make for difficulties in holding a particular line so far as people who are 'unloved, unlovely and unloveable' are concerned (Prins 1993b: 54). This acknowledgement of the hard facts about mentally disordered offending, and the preparedness not to shy away from it is important. Recognising – and naming the fact – that these individuals constitute a 'constantly shifting mad, bad and sad group' (Prins 1993a) is an important step in coming to terms with the sheer multi-dimensional complexity of what has to be faced in the management of these individuals (Stone 1995; Grant, and Preston-Shoot, this volume).

Offender, deviant or patient?[2]

A reminder of the bases upon which we ought to approach these of our fellow citizens is surely important, given the difficulties that they pose to those who are charged with their 'management'. Jill Peay has elsewhere argued 'that the mentally disordered offender be treated as a person first, as an offender second, and as mentally disordered third' (Peay 1994: 1123). But this is not just a set of ethical imperatives, designed to rescue a measure of humanity from the frequently hard to love, or an injunction to remember that mentally disordered offenders are not a homogeneous group. The three-way separation of attributes also refers to the three professional domains that are of relevance here. Social work, law and medicine (the last of these – doubtless unfairly – having to serve as a portmanteau term that covers those professions associated with medicine, and in particular mental health nursing) are in their different ways primarily responsible for respectively understanding the person-in-situation, for assessing the substance and culpability of their legal infraction, and for determining the mental conditions which might have lessened a capacity for rationality.

Inevitably, these domains are difficult to separate out, and while the contributors to this collection write within one or other framework, they inevitably stray beyond the boundaries of their discipline of preference. Indeed, this eclecticism has long marked the approach that Herschel Prins has himself adopted, pragmatically calling upon this or that body of knowledge to further the scope of his enquiry. What they have in common, though, is an attempt to ensure that the bases upon which the mentally disordered offender are judged ought to be consistent with various principles of justice and humanity. Eclecticism – sometimes derided for its lack of philosophical robustness – is warranted in an activity that draws its analytical blade across such alternating territory. Countenancing the possibility of a crime being rationally committed, alongside the equally feasible possibility of an incapacitated mind at work, invites a merging of categorical certainties about those who are mentally disordered and those who are not. There may indeed be shades of grey in the capacity behind all human motivation, suggesting that a measure of philosophical diffidence rather than the certitude of forensic science may – at least for some of the time – be the preferable way of approaching the waywardness of those who are mentally disordered. Hudson (1996: 156) draws on Levinas in offering an approach to justice which to our mind connects so well with what Herschel Prins (and the contributors to this *Festschrift*) are looking to secure – a balance between over-riding general principles and the particularities of individuals – that it can well stand as the final sentence to this collection:

> Justice is recognition of the Other, who is like myself in some ways, and unlike in others; justice involves recognition of the likeness in the sense of shared humanness, but not insistence on reduction or elimination of difference, rather the respecting of differences.
>
> (Hudson 1996: 15)

Notes

1 The 'civilising process' is a phrase borrowed (in rather cavalier fashion and with what is almost certainly insufficient regard to the conceptual sophistications of its origins) from the work of the sociologist Norbert Elias (1897–90). His concern was with the ways in which the coercive restraints of pre-modern society are superseded – or not – by moral obligation and the increasing awareness of the consequences that our actions have not only on the material circumstances of others but on the subjectivities of their minds too. The extent to which our treatment of the mentally disordered – whether offenders or not – exemplifies the process that Elias sought to demonstrate in his historical sociology is, of course, the matter at hand in this book. For those who find *ad hominem* things interesting, Norbert Elias's visiting professorship in the sociology Department at Leicester University overlapped with Herschel Prins's time at the School of Social Work at the same university. As far as I am aware they had no professional contact, though a resilient optimism and a sorely tested belief in humanity could be taken as a shared 'meta narrative' to their work, reflecting certain biographical commonalities.
2 This sub-heading is, of course, the same as that of one of Herschel Prins's books (Prins 1995). It summarises neatly the various 'discourses' which have something to say about the mentally disordered offender, the various roles to which these people can be assigned, and the endless possibilities for confusion about which in its more impatient moments, this book has made great play.

References

Busfield, J. (1996) *Men, Women and Madness: Understanding Gender and Mental Disorder* Basingstoke: Macmillan.

Craft, M. (1984) 'Who are mentally disordered offenders?' In M. Craft and A. Craft (eds) *Mentally Abnormal Offenders*. London: Ballière Tindall.

Donnelly, M. (1983) *Managing the Mind: A Study of Medical Psychology in Early Nineteenth Century Britain*. London: Tavistock.

Duff, A. and Garland, D. (eds) (1995) *A Reader in Punishment*. Oxford: Oxford University Press.

Halleck, S. (1987) *The Mentally Disordered Offender*. Washington, DC: American Psychiatric Press.

Higgins, J. (1994) *The Mentally Disordered Offender in his Society*. In M. Craft and A. Craft (eds) *Mentally Abnormal Offenders*. London: Ballière Tindall.

Hodgins, S. (1993) *Mental Disorder and Crime*. Newbury Park: Sage.

Hollin, C. and Howells, K. (1993) 'The mentally disordered offender: a clinical approach'. In K. Howells and C. Hollin (eds) *Clinical Approaches to the Mentally Disordered Offender*. Chichester: Wiley.

Hudson, B. (1996) *Understanding Justice: An Introduction to Ideas, Perspectives and Controversies in Modern Penal Theory*. Buckingham: Open University Press.

McConville, S. (1995) 'Local justice: the jail'. In N. Morris and D. Rothman (eds) *The Oxford Handbook of the Prison: The Practice of Punishment in Western Society*. Oxford: Oxford University Press.

Morris, N. (1995) '"Dangerousness" and incapacitation', in A. Duff and D. Garland (eds), *A Reader in Punishment*. Oxford: Oxford University Press.

Pearson, G. (1975) *The Deviant Imagination: Psychiatry, Social Work and Social Change*. London: Macmillan.

Peay, J. (1994) 'Mentally disordered offenders'. In M. Maguire, R. Morgan and R. Reiner (eds) *The Oxford Handbook of Criminology*. Oxford: Clarendon Press.

Prins, H. (1975) 'A danger to themselves and to others: social workers and potentially dangerous clients'. *British Journal of Social Work* 5 (3), 297–309.

—— (1983) 'Diminished responsibility and the Sutcliffe case: legal, psychiatric and social aspects'. *Medicine, Science and Law*, 23 (1), 17–24.

—— (1993a) 'Service provision and facilities for the mentally disordered offender'. In K. Howells and C. Hollin (eds) *Clinical Approaches to the Mentally Disordered Offender*. Chichester, Wiley.

—— (1993b) 'Offenders-patients: the people nobody owns'. In W. Watson and A. Grounds (eds) *The Mentally Disordered Offender in an Era of Community Care*. Cambridge: Cambridge University Press.

—— (Chairman) (1993c) *Report of the Committee of Enquiry into the Death in Broadmoor Hospital of Orville Blackwood and a Review of the Death of Two Other Afro-Caribbean Patients: 'Big, Black and Dangerous?'* London: Special Hospital Service Authority.

—— (1994) 'Is diversion just a diversion?' *Medicine, Science and Law* 34 (2), 137–147.

—— (1995) *Offenders, Deviants or Patients?* (rev. edn). London: Routledge.

Rotman, E. (1995) 'Beyond punishment'. In A. Duff and D. Garland (eds) *A Reader in Punishment*. Oxford: Oxford University Press.

Sedgewick, P. (1982) *PsychoPolitics*. London: Pluto Press.

Shah, S. (1993) 'A clinical approach to the mentally disordered offender: an overview and some major issues.' In K. Howells and C. Hollin (eds) *Clinical Approaches to the Mentally Disordered Offender*. Chichester: Wiley.

Stone, N. (1995) *A Companion Guide to Mentally Disordered Offenders*. Ilkley: Owen Wells.

Webb, D. (1976) 'Wise after the event: some comments on "A danger to themselves and others"', *British Journal of Social Work* 6 (1), 91–96.

Webster, C. and Menzies, R., 'Supervision in the de-institutionalised community'. In S. Hodgins (1993) *Mental Disorder and Crime*. Newbury Park: Sage.

Index

accountability, multiple 76–7
Ackroyd, P. 18
actuarial welfare 161–5
Adams, R. 77
Agass, D. 72, 77, 78, 88
Ancel, M. 22
'appropriate adults' (AAs) 39, 41, 44, 48
'approved social workers' (ASWs) 45, 46–7, 50, 85
Arms for Iraq Inquiry 32, 33
Ashworth Hospital Inquiry 28–31, 32, 33, 34, 35
assessment: needs-led 79; psychiatric 60, 61–7; risk *see* risk management
Association of Chief Officers of Probation 100
Atkinson, J. 84

bail 4, 58–9, 68, 69
Bail Act (1976) 69
Barclay Report 76, 86
Barker, A. 118
Barker, M. 96
Barnes, D. 73, 75, 80
Barnet Crisis Intervention Service 65–6
Baron, J. 148
Barry, N. 83
Bean, P. 3–4, 10, 38–51
Beckett, R. 100
Beckford, Jasmine 34
Ben-Yehuda, N. 95
Best, D. 85
black defendants 59, 161
Blackburn, R. 13, 14, 15
Blackwood Inquiry 27–8, 29, 30, 31, 32, 161
Bland, R. 85
Blaug, R. 81

Blom-Cooper, Louis 2, 27–36, 148, 49, 164
Bluglass, R. 44
Blumenthal, S. 65, 67–8
Bradley, C. 142
Braye, S. 75, 76, 77, 78, 80, 81, 85, 86
Brittain, Leon 112
Brixton Prison 56
Broadmoor Special Hospital 27–8, 29, 30, 31, 32, 33, 35
Brooke, D. 53, 54, 114
BSE Inquiry 33
Buckley, J. 73
Burney, E. 64
Busfield, J. 159, 163
Butler Committee Report 12, 42
Butler-Sloss, E. 75
Bynoe, I. 42

Canterbury and Thanet Community Healthcare Trust 66
care management 80
Care Programme Approach 72, 73, 76, 80
Carlile, Kimberley 34
Carpenter, J. 73, 76
Carson, D. 150
Casement, P. 72
categorization, problems of 14
Cavadino, P. 4, 5, 13, 53–70, 160
Cecchin, G. 72
Christie, N. 17
Clear, T. 99
Clerkenwell Magistrates' Court 61–2
Cleveland Report 75
Clunis, Christopher 76, 141, 144–5, 150–1
Cohen, S. 95
Commission on Social Justice 73
common good 22
communication, effective 145–8

community care 2, 5–6, 23, 68, 72–3, 80, 81
competence of organisations 87
consent to treatment 84
cooperation, multi-agency 5, 6, 43, 64–5, 95–110, 160
Copas, J.B. 114
cost of inquiries 33
court assessment schemes 61–5
Craft, A. 12
Craft, M. 12, 13, 158
Crichton, J. 142
Crighton, S. 114
Crime (Sentences) Act (1997) 79, 84
Criminal Evidence (Amendment) Act (1997) 79
Criminal Justice Act (1991) 60, 69, 112
criminality and mental disorder 11–13
Crown Prosecution Service 60
Cumming, I. 55
custody: diversion from 4, 59–70; impact of 54–6

Darnell, G. 28
Darvill, G. 90
Davies, N. 86
decision-making 148; by Mental Health Review Tribunals 132–3
dehumanisation 75–8
Department of Health 40, 42, 44, 47, 59, 65, 67, 75, 84, 85
diminished responsibility 12, 14, 16, 144
Disabled Persons Act (1986) 75–6
discrimination 90
Ditchfield, J. 114, 115, 123
diversion from custody 4, 59–70
Donnelly, M. 161
Donoghue v Stevenson [1932] 143
Dooley, E. 55–6
Drakeford, M. 77, 79
drug abuse 48–9
dual-diagnosis patients 48–9
Duff, A. 158, 163
Duncan, S. 143

Eastman, N. 150
Eaves, D. 114, 115, 124
Elias, N. 166n
empowerment 79, 82, 84–5, 88, 89
enhanced supervision 101–2
ethics 85, 88
European Convention on Human Rights and Fundamental Freedoms 76

fairness of inquiries 32, 34
families of victims 35
Faulkner, A. 40, 42, 43, 73, 75
Feldman, P. 12, 14
Fisher, D. 96
Fitzmaurice, C. 148, 149
Floud, J. 12
Forbes, J. 78
Freund, K. 104
fundamental attribution error 148, 149

Garland, D. 158, 163
Gerber, P. 12
Glueck, S. 12, 14, 21
Gobert, J. 152
Goddard, R. 34–5
Gomm, R. 85
Goode, E. 95
Gostin, L. 14–15
Grant, D. 5–6, 95–110, 160
Grimwood, C. 77
Grounds, A. 14, 36, 56–8
guardianship orders 60
Gunn, J. 12, 53

Halleck, S. 157, 159, 164
Hamilton, L. 61, 62
Harrington, G. 28
Harris, R. 1–9, 10–24, 99, 158
Hawkins, K. 148
Health, Department of 40, 42, 44, 47, 59, 65, 67, 75, 84, 85
Hedderman, C. 65
Heidensohn, F. 14
Henkel, M. 77, 84
The Herald of Free Enterprise 152
Herrnstein, R. 17
Higgins, J. 156–7
HM Prison Service 56
Hodgins, S. 160
Hoggett, B. 44
Hollin, C. 12, 164
Holloway Prison 56, 57
Home Office 12, 40, 42, 43, 46, 47, 56, 59, 61, 65, 66, 67, 69, 98, 115
homicide, inquiries after 142–3, 145–8
Hood, R. 113, 119, 122, 123
hospital orders 60, 61
hospital transfers, parole of 121–2
Howard, Michael 112
Howe, Lord 33
Howells, K. 164
Howlett, M. 72

Hudson, B. 157, 162, 166
Husband, C. 86
Hutton, W. 86

images of mentally disordered people
78–9, 89
imprisonment *see* custody
individuality, respect for 88–9
inquiries 2–3, 8, 27–36, 141, 148–50; after
homicide 142–3, 145–8; cost of 33;
fairness of 32, 34; legal representation
in 32, 33; private versus public 30, 31,
33–6, 164
insanity defence 12, 14–15
inter-agency working *see* multi-agency
cooperation
Irwin, S. 144
Islington Mentally Disordered Offenders
Project 64

James, A. 90
James, D. 61, 62
Jessel, D. 12
Jones, R. 39, 42, 47
Jones, S. 74, 83
Joseph, P. 62, 63
Joss, R. 74
judicial reviews 82
justice 18–21, 22, 157–8, 165–6

Kaganas, F. 80
Kemshall, H. 98
Kennedy, M. 58–9
'knew it all along effect' 148, 149
Krarup, H. 56

labelling theory 161
Lacey, M. 99
Laming, H. 13
law and attribution of negligence 143–5,
150–2
Law Commission 75
legal representation in public inquiries 32,
33
legalism 5; in policy 81–4
Lemert, E.M. 95
Leslie, A. 75, 77, 81, 84
licence conditions, psychiatric 121
Liebling, A. 56
Lingham, R. 145, 147
Luke Warm Luke Mental Health inquiry
(Scotland Report) 31, 35
Lunacy Act (1890) 39

McConville, S. 160
Mace, A. 13
McGuire, J. 97, 98
McWilliams, W. 99
Mair, G. 98
Major, J. 141
management, as a term 161–2
Mankoff, M. 95
Martin, M. 28, 29
May, T. 99
Menninger, K. 17
Mental Health Act (1959) 12, 39, 127
Mental Health Act (1983) 60, 80, 130;
Section 136 38–50 *passim*, 60
Mental Health Act Commission (1993) 39,
40, 41, 44, 47, 48
Mental Health Foundation 66, 73
Mental Health (Patients in the
Community) Act (1995) 72, 76, 84
Mental Health Review Tribunals 7–8,
127–40, 158
Mental Illness Specific Grant 73
Menzies, I. 77
Menzies, R. 162
MIND 41–2, 43
Mitchell, D. 76
Mitchell, Jason 34–5, 148, 149
M'Naghten Test 12
Moir, A. 12
Monahan, J. 145, 152
Morgan, R. 96
Morris, N. 163
Moulin, P. 10, 17
multi-agency cooperation 5, 6, 43, 64–7,
68, 83, 95–110, 160
multi-disciplinarity 3
Munro, E. 78, 84, 88
Mustill, M. 12

National Association for the Care and
Resettlement of Offenders (NACRO)
41, 59, 66
Needham-Bennett, H. 55
needs-led assessments 79
negligence 141, 143–5, 150–2, 164
Nemitz, T. 41, 44, 48
Newton, J. 73
NHS and Community Care Act (1990) 80
Norrie, A. 15
North Humberside Diversion Project 65

O'Leary, V. 99
Onyett, S. 77

organisations, competence of 87
'outlier' status of mentally disturbed 1, 4

Parkin, A. 76, 82, 83
parole 6–7, 158
Parole Board 6, 7, 112–25
partnership 74–5, 79, 84–5
Pearson, G. 64
Pease, K. 148, 149
Peay, J. 8, 16, 115, 124, 127, 128, 141–54,
   160, 162, 164, 165
Petch, E. 142
Pietroni, M. 79, 83
Pilgrim, D. 77, 81
Pinder, M. 13
Pitchers, J. 6–7, 112–25, 158, 159
Pithouse, A. 98
place of safety, removal to a 38–51, 60
police 3–4, 38–51
Police and Criminal Evidence Act (1984)
   (PACE) 41, 45, 46–7, 48
police stations, as places of safety 40–4,
   49–50
police surgeons 3–4, 45–6
policy-making and guidance 74–5, 79–80,
   87; legalism in 81–4
Popplestone, R. 77
Potter, M. 62, 63
power relationships 74–5, 88
Preston-Shoot, M. 4–5, 72–91, 160
Priestley, P. 98
Prins, Herschel 1, 11, 13, 15, 20, 34, 50,
   72, 74, 78, 79, 81, 82, 83, 86, 95, 115,
   141, 158, 160, 162, 165; on committees
   of inquiry 2, 27, 31, 33, 34, 36
Prior, P. 84, 89–90
probation 5–6
probation orders 60
probation service 60, 124–5; and
   management of sex offenders 98, 100,
   102–10
procedurally led practice 81–2
psychiatric assessment 60, 61–8, 115–16,
   117–19, 124, 129
psychiatric medicine 128–9
psychiatric panels 119–21
psychological reports 119
public inquiries see inquiries
purchaser/provider split 77

Radzinowicz, L. 14, 22
Rassaby, E. 43
Raynor, P. 98

reason and rationality 14, 15–19, 148–50
Reder, P. 75, 78, 81, 83, 143
Reed Report 40, 43, 47, 67, 68–9
rehabilitation of sex offenders 98–101
Reiner, R. 143
remand prisoners 53–4, 56–9, 60, 69
resources, lack of 76
responsibility 148–50, 164; diminished 12,
   14, 16, 144
Richardson, J.T. 95
rights versus risks 83, 88, 90
risk 72, 80, 83, 88, 90
risk management 5, 6–7, 8, 141, 163; of
   mentally disordered sex offenders
   95–110; and the Parole Board 112–25
Risk of Reconviction (RoR) score 114
Risley Prison 56
Ritchie, J. 73, 77, 81, 141, 150
Robbins, D. 75, 84
Roberts, C. 98
Rogers, A. 40, 41, 43, 77, 81
Rose, D. 79
Rotman, E. 164
Royal College of Psychiatrists 39, 41, 42,
   43, 46, 47, 118

Sandford, J. 83
Sashidharan, S. 78
Sbaraini, S. 73, 76
Scotland Report 31, 35
Scott Inquiry into Arms for Iraq 32, 33
Sedgewick, P. 161
Seedhouse, D. 86
self-determination 90
self-harm 54, 55–6
sentencing 60
Sex Offender Risk Management Approach
   (SORMA) 6, 102–10
sex offenders 5–6, 95–110, 120
Shah, S. 158, 163
Shaw, G.B. 11, 20
Sheppard, D. 73, 75, 76, 77, 142
Shorter, E. 128
Shute, S. 113, 119, 122, 123
Sinclair Inquiry 145–8
social labelling 161
social order and mental disorder 10–24
social work 4–5, 72–91
staff: dehumanisation of 75–8; support and
   supervision of 78
Staite, C. 13, 65
Steele, G. 28
stereotyping 78, 89

substance misuse 48–9, 53–4
suicide 54, 55–6
supervised discharge orders 72, 82
supervision registers 72, 82
supervision of staff 78
surveillance 6
Sutcliffe, Peter 12, 160
Szasz, T. 128

Tawney, R.H. 19
therapy for sex offenders 97
Tidmarsh, D. 147
Timms, N. 13, 18
Turner, J. 14

values 5; for practice 84–6
Vass, A.A. 99
victims, families of 35
violence 79, 115, 124

Walton, P. 77
Walton, S. 28
Wardhaugh, J. 75
Watts, J. 28, 29
Webb, D. 1–9, 82, 83, 156–66
Webster, C. 162
Webster, C.D. 114, 115, 124
Wessely, S. 65, 67–8
West, D.J. 112
Wilding, P. 75
Wilson, G. 73
Wilson, J.Q. 17
Wood, J. 7–8, 127–40, 158

Yelloly, M. 77, 83
Young, J. 95, 100, 102
Young, W. 12

Zito, J. 72, 141